# FIRST AID FOR THE MATCH

## INSIDER ADVICE FROM STUDENTS AND RESIDENCY DIRECTORS

**2nd Edition**

**TAO LE, MD**
*University of California, San Francisco, Class of 1996*
*Founder and Chief Medical Officer, Medschool.com*

**VIKAS BHUSHAN, MD**
*University of California, San Francisco,*
*Class of 1991*
*Founder and CEO, Medschool.com*

**CHIRAG AMIN, MD**
*University of Miami, Class of 1996*
*Vice President, Community and Content,*
*Medschool.com*

**McGraw-Hill**
Medical Publishing Division

New York   St. Louis   San Francisco   Auckland   Bogotá   Caracas   Lisbon   London
Madrid   Mexico City   Milan   Montreal   New Delhi   San Juan
Singapore   Sydney   Tokyo   Toronto

## McGraw-Hill

*A Division of The* **McGraw·Hill** *Companies*

ISBN: 0-8385-2607-1
ISSN: 1090-364X

---

### Notice

Medicine is an ever-changing science. As new research and clinical experience broaden our knowledge,
changes in treatment and drug therapy are required. The authors and the publisher of this work have
checked with sources believed to be reliable in their efforts to provide information that is complete and
generally in accord with the standards accepted at the time of publication. However, in view of the
possibility of human error or changes in medical sciences, neither the authors nor the publisher nor any
other party who has been involved in the preparation or publication of this work warrants that the
information contained herein is in every respect accurate or complete, and they disclaim all responsibility
for any errors or omissions or for the results obtained from use of the information contained in this work.
Readers are encouraged to confirm the information contained herein with other sources. For example and
in particular, readers are advised to check the product information sheet included in the package of each
drug they plan to administer to be certain that the information contained in this work is accurate and that
changes have not been made in the recommended dose or in the contraindications for administration. This
recommendation is of particular importance in connection with new or infrequently used drugs.

---

This book was set in Goudy by Rainbow Graphics.
The editors were Shelley Reinhardt and Isabel Nogueira.
The production supervisor was Phil Galea.
Production management was provided by Rainbow Graphics.

Courier Kendallville was printer and binder.

This book is printed on acid-free paper.

To the contributors to this and future editions,
who took time to share their experience,
advice, and humor for the benefit of students.

&

To our families, friends, and loved ones,
who endured and assisted in the task of assembling this guide.

# Contributors

**DARREN DON, MD**
University of California, Los Angeles,
School of Medicine, Class of 2000
Good Samaritan Hospital,
Resident in Internal Medicine

**ROSS LEVINE, MD**
Johns Hopkins University, School of Medicine
Class of 1999
Massachusetts General Hospital,
Resident in Internal Medicine

**MICHELLE PINTO, MD**
Yale University School of Medicine, Class of 1999
Brigham and Women's Hospital,
Resident in Internal Medicine

**DEBORAH STEINBAUM, MD**
Yale University School of Medicine, Class of 1999
The Mount Sinai Hospital, New York,
Resident in Pediatrics/Primary Care

**NINA EISENBERG, MD**
Yale University School of Medicine, Class of 1999
Montefiore Medical Center,
Resident in Psychiatry

**KEN LIN, MD**
University of California, Los Angeles, School of Medicine,
Class of 2000
Cedars-Sinai Medical Center,
Resident in Internal Medicine/Pediatrics

**JEANNINE RAHIMIAN, MD, MBA**
University of California, Los Angeles, School of Medicine,
Class of 2000
UCLA Medical Center,
Resident in Obstetrics and Gynecology

# Contents

# Foreword

There are predictable times in the course of medical education that will engender in nearly every student some combination of excitement, anxiety, and dread. The *First Aid* series aims to assist students through these times by providing sound, thoughtful, student-oriented guidance and advice, and *First Aid for the Match* continues this tradition. *First Aid for the USMLE Step 1* has fulfilled these goals and has reached an audience of more than 80,000 medical students in five years.

As Dean of Students at a distinguished school of medicine for a number of years, I had the pleasure of working with over a thousand medical students in their passage through the exercises of career choice, residency selection, and negotiation of the challenges of the "Match." I was responsible for writing all of their deans' letters—letters seen by both the subjects and the recipients as having both critical importance and dubious value. Each student brought to the process their hopes and fears, their pride and their (sometimes not very hidden) insecurities. There is no doubt that the choice of specialty and the choice of residency program are of major consequence. Yet faculty advisers and student affairs deans are rarely entirely up to the task of providing students facing these choices with the information and advice called for. And not surprisingly, students often wonder whether the advice being given is to some degree driven by the faculty's own concerns and wishes rather than entirely in the students' interests.

*First Aid for the Match* provides its readers with much of the key facts and advice needed to work through this process. It cannot and should not substitute for the valuable advice and counsel that students can best receive from faculty advisers and members of the dean's staff. And it cannot replace the currency of "word of mouth" information received from student colleagues and residents who have recently survived these challenges. However, it successfully supplements these sources with recent, verified data about residency selection, up-to-date information about the various core residency training specialties, helpful tips on selecting both specialties and residencies, and useful guidance concerning such critical events as writing a personal statement, being interviewed, and succeeding in the match process itself.

The essence of this process is that every party involved is hoping for the best possible results. The residency program certainly wants to acquire an outstanding new crop of house staff, to maintain the program's pride, to provide assurance that faculty will be well challenged by the best and brightest, and to ensure that patients will receive the best possible medical care. The medical school wants to ensure that its graduates achieve their highest choices, both for its own pride and traditions and so that incoming students can be assured that they will be well taken care of at the other end of their medical school experience. Lastly, and for whom this book is written, are the students going through the match process who see this as a critical step that can determine their future professional happiness and success.

How many of these goals are actually achieved certainly varies from program to program, school to school, and student to student. How many of those hoped-for results are actually determined by the Match is also not clear. What is certain is that students armed with current information resources such as *First Aid for the Match* generally do better in the residency application process.

The authors are anxious for your feedback and are committed to maintaining the currency of this book through these times of rapid change. I wish all the readers of this guide and all those going through the process of the Match the very best of luck and professional and personal success.

David F. Altman, M.D.
Associate Dean of Medical Students, 1982–1989
University of California, San Francisco

# Preface to the First Edition

Going through the residency application process can be a confusing, time-consuming, even hazardous adventure. If you make the right decisions, you will most likely find a residency position that suits you best. A bad or uninformed decision can derail your career and waste years of your life. The purpose of *First Aid for the Match* is to help medical students effectively and efficiently navigate the residency application process. This book helps students make the most of their limited time, money, and energy. In the spirit of *First Aid for the USMLE Step 1*, this book is a student-to-student guide that draws on the advice and experiences of medical students who have successfully gone through the Match and are now training in the programs of their choice. *First Aid for the Match* has a number of unique features that make it indispensable to the residency applicant:

- Insider advice from medical students and residency program directors.
- The latest trends in the residency application process and specialty fields.
- Application and interview tips tailored to each specialty.
- Real personal statements and résumés that worked.
- A student-tested guide to cheap, efficient interview travel and lodging.
- Common interview questions with suggested strategies for responding to each.
- Emergency protocols for the Scramble (if you do not match).
- A master checklist for the application process.

*First Aid for the Match* is meant to be a guide rather than a comprehensive source of information. It should supplement information and advice provided by other students, your adviser, and your dean's office. Though the material has been reviewed by medical faculty and students, errors and omissions are inevitable. We urge readers to suggest improvements and identify inaccuracies. We invite students and faculty to continue sharing their thoughts and ideas to help us improve *First Aid for the Match* (see How to Contribute, p. xix).

Santa Monica, CA                                             Tao Le, MD
Santa Monica, CA                                         Chirag Amin, MD
Santa Monica, CA                                       Vikas Bhushan, MD

October, 2000

# Preface

With the second edition of *First Aid for the Match,* we continue our commitment to providing students with the most useful and up-to-date information to help guide them through the residency application and interview process and obtain a residency position in the specialty of their choice. The second edition represents a thorough revision and includes:

- The latest insider advice from students who have successfully made it through the 2000 National Residency Matching Program (NRMP) Match
- Up-to-date information and statistics from the 2000 NRMP Match, including the latest trends in each of the specialty fields
- Expanded specialty coverage, with detailed information on 19 specialties, including neurosurgery, urology, and physical medicine and rehabilitation
- New information on the recently implemented Electronic Residency Application Service (ERAS), the web-based Rank Order List and the Input Confirmation System (ROLIC)
- Sample personal statements for each specialty
- Detailed listings of resources available over the Internet
- A completely revised, in-depth travel advice section (Chapter 8), with detailed information on discount airfares and hotel lodging, as well as descriptions of over 40 unique online travel and lodging sites
- An extensive compilation of commonly asked interview questions, broken down by specialty

The second edition would not have been possible without the help of a handful of dedicated students and faculty members who contributed their feedback and suggestions. We invite both students and faculty to share their thoughts and ideas to help us continue to improve *First Aid for the Match* in the future. (See How to Contribute, p. xix, and User Survey, p. xxiii.)

Santa Monica, CA                                                          Tao Le, MD
Santa Monica, CA                                                    Chirag Amin, MD
Santa Monica, CA                                                  Vikas Bhushan, MD

December 2000

# Acknowledgments

We owe special thanks to Dr. Lawrence Tierney, Dr. Stephen McPhee, Dr. Helen Loesser, Dr. Anthony Glaser, Dr. Eric Schulze, Thao Pham, Dr. Daniel Lowenstein, Dr. Denise Rodgers, Dr. Linda Ferrell, Dr. Richard Odom, Dr. Patricia Robertson, Uzma Samadani, Esther Choo, Marinita Timban, David Steensma, Dr. Lisa Alsta, Dr. Daniela Drake, Dr. Sana Khan, and the UCSF School of Medicine Office of Student Affairs for their thoughtful comments, corrections, and advice.

Thanks to our editors Shelley Reinhardt and Catherine Johnson for their enthusiasm, support, and commitment to the First Aid books. Thanks to Christie Nagleri and Isabel Nogueira for their tireless administrative assistance. For support and encouragement throughout the process, we are grateful to Gianni Nguyen and Jonathan Kirsch.

For submitting feedback and contributions, we thank David Anick, Perry Brown, Carrie Chen, Antony Chu, Eddie Frothingham, Anna Hejinian, Tony Hill, Catherine Hoffman, Peter Hofmann, Clara Hsu, Bruce Lattyak, Mark Lee, Rick Miller, Sonia Nagy, Elizabeth Oudens, Rajiv Rathod, Kelly Ray, Noel Saks, Dennis Shay, Jacque Slaughter, Lisa Strate, Mel Stone, Judy Tjoe, and Margo Vener.

# How to Contribute

*First Aid for the Match* incorporates many contributions and changes from students and faculty. We invite you to participate in this process.

Please send us:

- Strategies for applying and interviewing in your specialty.
- Your personal statement and CV (feel free to edit or mask for privacy).
- Anecdotes of your application and interviewing experiences.
- Your medical school's guide to the Match.
- Corrections and clarifications.

Personalized contributions (i.e., anecdotes and personal statements), if used, will be altered to protect the identity of the contributor. For each entry incorporated into the next edition, you will receive a personal acknowledgment in the next edition. Significant contributions will be compensated at the discretion of the authors.

The preferred way to submit suggestions and corrections is via electronic mail, addressed to:

**FirstAidMatch@medschool.com**

For *First Aid for the Match* updates and corrections, visit our Book Errata section (under Discussion Forums, or locate it via the Site Map) Internet website at:

**http://students.medschool.com**

Otherwise, please send entries, neatly written or typed or on disk (Microsoft Word), to: **First Aid for the Match, 1015 Gayley Ave., #1113, Los Angeles, CA 90024, Attention: Contributions.** Please use the contribution and survey forms on the following pages. Each form constitutes an entry. (Attach additional pages as needed.

Another option is to send in your entire annotated book. We will look through your additions and notes and will send you an honorarium based on the quantity and quality of any additions that we incorporate into the next edition. Books will be returned upon request. Contributions sent earlier will receive priority consideration for the next edition of *First Aid for the Match*.

## Internship Opportunities

The author team of Le, Amin, and Bhushan is pleased to offer part-time and full-time paid internships in medical education and publishing to motivated medical students and physicians. Internships may range from two to three months (e.g., a summer) up to a full year. Participants will have an opportunity to author, edit, and earn academic credit on a wide variety of projects, including the popular *First Aid* series. Writing/editing experience, familiarity with Microsoft Word, and Internet access are desired. For more information, e-mail a résumé or a short description of your experience along with a cover letter to FirstAidMatch@medschool.com.

## Note to Contributors

All entries are subject to editing and reviewing. Please verify all data and spellings carefully. In the event that similar or duplicate entries are received, only the first entry received will be used. Please follow the style, punctuation, and format of this edition if possible.

# Contribution Form

For tips and strategies for
applying and interviewing
in your specialty.

Contributor Name: _____

School/Affiliation: _____

Address: _____

_____

Telephone: _____

_____

**Your specialty:** _____

Type of program where you matched:  __ Clinical
__ Academic

Region where you applied (e.g., Northeast, both coasts): _____

_____

Application trends in your specialty:




_____

Application tips for your specialty:




_____

Interview tips for your specialty:




_____

Specialty resources (e.g., useful books, articles, directories on the specialty):




_____

Other comments:

*Please return by April 15th following the Match. You will receive personal acknowledgment for material used in future editions.*

(fold here)

Return Address

_____

_____

_____

**BUSINESS REPLY MAIL**
FIRST-CLASS MAIL PERMIT NO. 74036 LOS ANGELES CA

POSTAGE WILL BE PAID BY ADDRESSEE

**FIRST AID FOR THE MATCH**
**1015 GAYLEY AVE. #1113**
**LOS ANGELES CA 90024-8980**

(fold here)

# User Survey

Contributor Name: _____

School/Affiliation: _____

Address: _____

_____

Telephone: _____

What student-to-student advice would you give someone going through the application process?

What would you change about the specialty overviews, application tips, interviewing tips, and specialty resources in Chapter 3?

What would you change about the application, personal statement, and CV tips?

What travel and interviewing tips would you change or add?

Is there an interesting application or interviewing experience that you would like to share?

How else would you improve *First Aid for the Match*? Any comments or suggestions? What did you like most about the book?

**Please return by April 15th following the Match. You will receive personal acknowledgment for material used in future editions.**

---------------------------------- (fold here) ----------------------------------

**Return Address**

_____

_____

_____

IIII

**BUSINESS REPLY MAIL**
FIRST-CLASS MAIL PERMIT NO. 74036 LOS ANGELES CA

POSTAGE WILL BE PAID BY ADDRESSEE

**FIRST AID FOR THE MATCH**
**1015 GAYLEY AVE. #1113**
**LOS ANGELES CA 90024-8980**

II.I..II...II.....I.I.I..II.I..II.I.I..I.I..II...II...I

---------------------------------- (fold here) ----------------------------------

# The Match

## INTRODUCTION

Relax.

This chapter will help to familiarize you with the Match. Our goal is to minimize your stress, maximize the fruits of your efforts, and improve your chances of landing an optimal residency position. As a medical student, you undoubtedly remember the process of medical school applications and interviews. However, the Match has different rules and strategies. The entire process can be overwhelming; each year, some students end up in an unsatisfactory program or unmatched, wondering what went wrong on Match Day. It is easy to lose sight of your goals and not obtain the residency position you desire. And since most students go through the Match only once, mistakes can lead to a lifetime of regret.

The Match is a giant "computer dating game" of sorts. But the fact that this relationship is an intimate one that lasts for 3 years or more means you need to ensure that your potential partner has compatible goals and interests. Conversely, directors of residency programs are searching for the best students. Therefore, you must know the right moves and when to make them. Asking how much the pay is for a resident is akin to asking a date his or her weight. You may be dying to know, but discretion is key.

Of course, the two biggest fears are (1) not matching at any program; and (2) ending up in a program that makes you miserable. Approximately 6.1% of U.S. students, 31.9% of Canadian participants and 61.5% of the non-U.S. foreign graduates in the National Residency Matching Program (NRMP) were "stood up" on the big day in 2000. Conversely, over 10% of available NRMP positions remained unfilled. Common mistakes that students make when going through the Match process include the following:

> ASKING HOW MUCH THE PAY IS FOR A RESIDENT IS AKIN TO ASKING A DATE HIS OR HER WEIGHT.

- ▶ Not understanding the details of the Match for a particular specialty
- ▶ Starting the application process too late
- ▶ Applying to or ranking too few programs to ensure a match
- ▶ Letting the application paperwork overwhelm you
- ▶ Ignoring key NRMP publications
- ▶ Submitting a weak personal statement and curriculum vitae
- ▶ Not knowing what to look for in a residency training program
- ▶ Preparing inadequately for residency interviews

> ▶ Ranking programs on the basis of probability of acceptance rather than desirability
>
> ▶ Panicking after failing to match, rather than intelligently playing the "Scramble"

In this chapter, we will help you understand the Match to guard you against these common pitfalls.

## WHAT IS THE MATCH?

Although there are actually several matches, most people know the NRMP as **the** Match. Although the NRMP offers positions in a wide range of specialties, there are some specialties that use their own match such as neurology, neurosurgery, ophthalmology, otolaryngology, and urology (Table 1–1). With over 90% of all graduating U.S. and Canadian medical students participating, as well as a surprisingly high number of international medical graduates, the NRMP is the largest match by far (Figure 1–1).

The basic modus operandi of the Match is as follows. After the interview season, residency training programs submit a list of applicants in the order in which they would offer acceptances; students enter lists of programs in the order in which they would accept offers. Both students and programs submit their rankings to the NRMP. Then, in a matter of minutes, a computer program matches the student to the highest program on his or her list that offered a position. The Match usually occurs in late February; the results are then announced simultaneously across the country on "Match Day" in mid-March. In 2000, 33,528 applicants enrolled in the Match, of the 25,056 applicants who submitted rank lists, 18,391 received offers (Figure 1–2). This

| TABLE 1–1. Specialties with their own matches. | | | |
|---|---|---|---|
| **Specialty** | **Matching Program** | **Month of Match Day** | **Website** |
| Neurology | Neurology Matching Program<br>P.O. Box 7999<br>San Francisco, CA 94120<br>(415) 923-3907 | January of senior year | http://www.sfmatch.org |
| Neurosurgery | Neurosurgical Surgery Matching Program<br>P.O. Box 7999<br>San Francisco, CA 94120<br>(415) 923-3907 | January of senior year | http://www.sfmatch.org |
| Ophthalmology | Ophthalmology Matching Program<br>P.O. Box 7999<br>San Francisco, CA 94120<br>(415) 923-3907 | January of senior year | http://www.sfmatch.org |
| Otolaryngology | Otolaryngology Matching Program<br>P.O. Box 7999<br>San Francisco, CA 94120<br>(415) 923-3907 | January of senior year | http://www.sfmatch.org |
| Urology | AUA Residency Matching Program<br>2425 West Loop South<br>Suite 333<br>Houston, TX 77027-4207<br>(713) 622-2700, ext: 86<br>Fax: (713) 622-2898 | Late January of senior year | http://www.avanet.org |

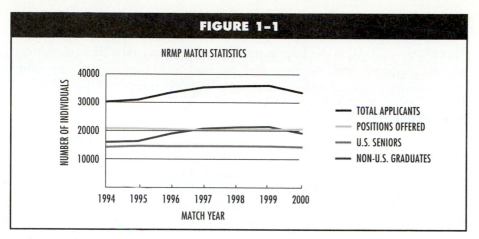

FIGURE 1-1

NRMP MATCH STATISTICS

NUMBER OF INDIVIDUALS

40000

30000

20000

10000

—— TOTAL APPLICANTS
—— POSITIONS OFFERED
—— U.S. SENIORS
—— NON-U.S. GRADUATES

1994  1995  1996  1997  1998  1999  2000

MATCH YEAR

Applicants in the NRMP Match.

translates into an overall match rate of 69.5% into a PGY-1 residency program.

If you are a U.S. medical student, you automatically receive information about the NRMP Match through your school in the spring of your third year. However, the NRMP can be contacted directly for more information at:

National Residency Matching Program
2450 N Street NW, Suite 201
Washington, DC 20037-1141
(202) 828-0676 for U.S. seniors
(202) 828-0566 for independent applicants
http://www.aamc.org/nrmp

## WHY IS THERE A MATCH?

By the late 1940s, the traditional matching process was growing increasingly chaotic. There were almost twice as many residency positions as there were U.S. medical graduates. More competitive programs had the luxury of receiving and reviewing large batches of applications before doling out their residency spots late in the students' fourth year. Less competitive programs tried to get a head start by asking students to commit to the program early in the fourth year or even during the third year.

As a result, students were forced to gamble by deciding whether to accept an early offer from a less competitive program and forfeit a later shot at better programs or to pass up the early offer and risk not being accepted in a better program. Residency directors faced a similar dilemma. If they filled all their positions too early, they would not be able to offer a position to a more desirable candidate who applied later; however, if they held out for better applicants, they risked not filling their programs.

As a solution to these dilemmas, the first Match was held in 1952. It was a huge success, with over 98% of the residency programs and 97% of the students participating. The Match eliminated guessing games for the most part by allowing applicants and programs to rank each other on the basis of desirability. The algorithm used to match applicants with programs has remained largely unchanged over the years. For a simple explanation of how the matching algorithm works, see Chapter 10.

FIGURE 1-2

33,528
enrolled

25,056
rank lists

20,598
PGY-1 positions
available

18,391
matched (69.5%)

Flowchart of the NRMP Match, based on 2000 NRMP Match data.

## WHAT OTHER MATCHES ARE THERE?

Though the NRMP is the largest matching program available to American medical students and international medical graduates, there are other matches as well, including some that operate independently of the NRMP.

### Specialties With Their Own Matches

Some specialties have their own match processes with different match days. These specialties include neurology, ophthalmology, otolaryngology, and urology. Except for urology, these specialty matches are run by Dr. August Colenbrander, an ophthalmologist in San Francisco. Since many of these specialties require training in medicine, pediatrics, or surgery, most applicants also match through the NRMP for 1 or 2 years of transitional training before starting their specialty work. Many students aiming for these specialties also apply for another specialty in the NRMP Match as a backup (eg, general surgery as a backup for neurosurgery). Please refer to "Your Specialty and the Match" (pg. 23) for more specific matching information regarding your target specialty.

### NRMP Couples Match

ANY TWO PEOPLE CAN APPLY AS A COUPLE.

In the couples match, the NRMP allows any two people to be matched with residency programs in the same geographic area if they so desire. Any two people can apply as a couple. Partners apply and interview separately at programs in the same geographic region. They then submit a rank-order list of pairs of programs in the order in which they would accept offers. Because couples are often limited by geography, they often submit more applications to maximize the likelihood of a successful match. To help matters more, the rank-order list gives a couple the option of seeking matches in separate locations or allowing one partner to go unmatched if a couples match is not possible.

COUPLES MAY HAVE SOME ADVANTAGES OVER OTHER APPLICANTS IN THE MATCH.

Some residency directors and deans believe that many couples do better together in the Match than if they were to apply and match separately. Couples tend to be viewed as more stable and less likely to leave residency programs. Because of the hassles of moving again after residency, especially with kids, couples are more likely to contribute to the faculty pool of the institution where they trained. If a couple targets a program in the same specialty and one partner is more desirable, the residency selection will often move the less competitive partner higher on the rank-order list rather than dropping the more competitive partner (though the reverse can occur). In short, couples may have advantages in the Match, though it's probably no reason to start a relationship! Internship will be tough enough as is. For more information about the couples match, consult the section on "Special Cases" in your *NRMP Handbook for Students*.

### Shared-Schedule Match

Shared-schedule positions in the NRMP Match allow two people to share the duties and responsibilities of one residency position. An applicant enrolls individually in the NRMP Match and then pairs up with a partner (eg, a significant other) by completing a *Shared Residency Pair Form*, due in the fall preceding Match Day. The pair shares one NRMP applicant code, applies and interviews together, and submits a single rank-order list. Though each person spends less than full time working (eg, alternate months on rotation), both will spend more time in residency and will eventually do as much if not more work than a full-time resident. Many applicants seek shared-schedule positions because of family responsibilities or research, among other reasons. Consult "Special Cases" in your *NRMP Handbook for Students* for more information.

## Canadian Match

The Canadian Residency Matching Service (CaRMS) was founded in 1970. Like its U.S. counterpart, the CaRMS Match is an orderly approach to matching applicants to their top choices and residency programs to their preferred applicants. In fact, CaRMS uses the same matching algorithm as the NRMP. CaRMS Match Day is also in mid-March. Approximately 1500 Canadian students apply for about 1500 slots annually offered through the Canadian Match. CaRMS is open to U.S. seniors, though few apply. For more information, contact:

> Canadian Residency Matching Service
> 151 Slater Street, Suite 802
> Ottawa, Ontario, Canada K1P 5H3
> (613) 237-0075
> (800) 291-3727
> Fax: (613) 563-2860
> http://www.carms.ca

## Osteopathic Match

The Intern Registration Program, the osteopathic version of the Match, is run by the National Matching Services (NMS). All osteopathic graduates are required to take a 1-year osteopathic rotating internship approved by the American Osteopathic Association (AOA) before entering an osteopathic residency. Applicants interview in late summer and fall, submit a rank-order list by early January, and await results on the osteopathic Match Day in late January.

About 2200 osteopathic internships and 1100 residency positions are offered through the osteopathic match every year. Osteopathic residency directors have recently had more difficulty filling their positions, as osteopathic graduates have gained wider acceptance in allopathic residency programs and the AOA has relaxed its restrictions on osteopathic graduates pursuing allopathic training through the NRMP Match.

For more information, contact:

American Osteopathic Association
Department of Education
142 E. Ontario Street
Chicago, IL 60611
Phone (800) 621-1773, ext 7426
http://www.am-osteo-assn.org

National Matching Service
Box 1208
Lewiston, NY 14092-8208
Phone (716) 282-4013
Fax (716) 282-0611

National Matching Service
595 Bay Street, Suite 300
Toronto, Ontario, Canada M5G 2C2
Phone (416) 977-3431
Fax (416) 977-5020

## Armed Forces Match

Army, Navy, and Air Force residencies have their own matching process early in the senior year, several months earlier than the NRMP Match. Applicants usually have military service obligations (eg, graduates of Uniformed Services University of the Health Sciences School of Medicine and participants in the Health Professions Scholarship Program). After senior-year applicants have been interviewed, the military programs convene in late November and early December each year in a week-long affair known as "Selection Boards" to match programs and applicants. The nonmatch rate varies widely among the different services; nevertheless, simultaneous enrollment in the NRMP Match is highly recommended. All medical graduates of the Uniformed Services University are preferentially placed through an Armed Forces match. If you match with a military residency program, you are obliged to withdraw from the NRMP Match or from any other civilian match.

For more information on the Army military match, contact the regional AMEDD counselor.

For more information on the Air Force military match, contact:

Headquarters AFMPC/DPAME
550 C Street West, Suite 27
Randolph AFB, TX 78150-4729
(800) 531-5800
DSN 487-6331

For more information on the Navy military match, contact:

Bureau of Medicine and Surgery
Code 512
Washington, DC 20372-5300
(202) 653-1318

## WHAT ARE MY CHANCES OF SUCCESS IN THE MATCH?

In general, U.S. seniors do well in the NRMP Match. About 85% of U.S. seniors obtain one of their first three choices each year (Table 1–2). The U.S. senior nonmatch rate has held steady at 6 to 7% for the past 10 years. In contrast, other applicants fare rather poorly (Table 1–3): In the 2000 Match,

| Choice Obtained | Percent of U.S. Seniors (1995) | Percent of U.S. Seniors (1996) | Percent of U.S. Seniors (1997) | Percent of U.S. Seniors (1998) | Percent of U.S. Seniors (1999) | Percent of U.S. Seniors (2000) |
|---|---|---|---|---|---|---|
| First | 59.8 | 59.8 | 59.4 | 58.4 | 60.9 | 62.3 |
| Second | 15.6 | 15.7 | 16.0 | 16.4 | 15.7 | 15.3 |
| Third | 8.8 | 8.3 | 9.3 | 9.3 | 8.8 | 8.6 |
| Fourth | 5.5 | 5.8 | 5.3 | 5.7 | 5.5 | 4.7 |
| > Fourth | 10.0 | 10.3 | 10.2 | 10.2 | 9.3 | 9.1 |
| Unmatched | 7.3 | 7.9 | 7.3 | 6.5 | 6.2 | 6.1 |

TABLE 1–2. Success of U.S. Seniors in the NRMP Match.

only one-half of the U.S. graduates (as opposed to U.S. seniors) and international medical graduates (IMGs) in the NRMP were successfully matched. IMGs, whether U.S. citizens or not, generally fare the worst. Foreign national IMGs in particular have experienced significant declines in match rates, from 63.4% in 1991 to 38.5% in 2000.

## HOW DO I REGISTER FOR THE NRMP MATCH?

### U.S. Seniors

In the spring of your third year of medical school, you will receive a preprinted student agreement form to review and sign. Make sure that the name listed on the agreement matches the name you use on your residency applications. The current registration fee is $40, payable to the NRMP, and is nonrefundable. Upon registering, you will be assigned an NRMP Applicant Code that you will use to identify yourself on residency applications and correspondence. The deadline for registration is in July at the start of your senior year. Consult the current edition of the *NRMP Handbook for Students* for additional registration details.

### U.S. Graduates

If you graduated from a U.S. medical school accredited through the Liaison Committee for Medical Education (LCME), you can register through your own school or another U.S. medical school. You can also enroll directly with the NRMP as an Independent Applicant (see below). If you are sponsored by a U.S. medical school, the school will serve as your NRMP "home base," from which to submit your rank-order list and where you will receive NRMP correspondence, including your Match results. Your *Agreement for Students or Sponsored Graduates* must be signed by both you and the dean of student affairs at your sponsor school. Your nonrefundable registration fee is also $40. Upon registering, you will receive an NRMP Applicant Code used to identify yourself on residency applications and in correspondence. The deadline for registering is in October before Match Day. See the current edition of the *NRMP Handbook for Students* for registration details. Also visit the NRMP website at http://www.aamc.org/nrmp.

### Independent Applicants

The category of "independent applicants" includes several different groups: nonsponsored U.S. graduates, Canadian students/graduates, osteopathic students/graduates, and international medical graduates (IMGs). For information, contact the NRMP at (202) 828-0566 during the summer before the Match to receive the *NRMP Handbook for Independent Applicants*. Or, you can visit the NRMP website at http://www.aamc.org/nrmp. To enroll, submit a completed *Independent Applicant Agreement* and $90, payable to the NRMP. The NRMP might also independently verify or request to see your credentials in order to approve your Match eligibility status. For example, IMGs need to pass the USMLE Step 1 and 2 as well as the English Test to participate in the Match.

Following registration, you will be assigned an NRMP Applicant Code, which you will use to identify yourself on residency applications and in correspondence. You will also receive a confidential Personal Identification Number (PIN). Match results will be made available to independent appli-

| Applicant Type | PGY-1 Match Rate |
|---|---|
| **TABLE 1–3. 2000 NRMP Match rate.** | |
| U.S. seniors | 93.9% |
| Canadian students | 68.1% |
| U.S. graduates | 48.6% |
| Osteopaths | 71.6% |
| U.S. citizen foreign graduates | 51.4% |
| Non-U.S. foreign graduates | 38.5% |

cants during Match week via the web (http://www.aamc.org/nrmp) as well as through the NRMP Voice Response System (VRS) by calling (202) 828-0566. The registration deadline is in October before Match Day. Consult the current edition of the *NRMP Handbook for Independent Applicants* and visit the NRMP website (http://www.aamc.org/nrmp) for further details.

## WHAT ABOUT THE OTHER MATCHES?

If you are a U.S. medical student, information pamphlets and registration materials for specialties outside the NRMP Match should be available at your dean's office. Otherwise, you can contact the specialty match programs directly for information and registration forms (Table 1–1). To register for the Armed Forces Match, contact your military branch's Medical Personnel Counselor or your local Armed Forces recruitment officer. Don't forget to register for the NRMP Match regardless of what other matches you enroll in. There is nothing to prevent you from enrolling in multiple matches; you just can't accept more than one appointment. Many of the non-NRMP matches require a preliminary transitional year obtained through the NRMP Match. In addition, many of these matches are very competitive, and the NRMP Match is a nice backup. It's better to register, match in advance, and lose the $40 fee than to be unable to participate in the Match at all.

## NRMP PUBLICATIONS

The NRMP offers a slew of valuable publications that few students know about and fewer still take the time to read. A handbook and the *NRMP Directory* are distributed to every applicant upon registration. The rest can be ordered from the NRMP by calling (202)828-0416 or by filling out the NRMP Publications Order Form found in the back of the *NRMP Directory* and mailing it to:

> ATTN: Membership and Publication Orders
> National Residency Matching Program
> 2450 N Street, NW
> Washington, DC 20037-1129

You can also order NRMP publications through the NRMP website at http://www.aamc.org/nrmp. For each NRMP publication listed below, we include a list price, a description, and a rating based on utility.

## NRMP Handbook for Students

This handbook is available free of charge through U.S. medical schools and is for U.S. seniors and sponsored graduates. Read it from cover to cover. It describes the NRMP and its role in the residency application process. You will be able to decipher the NRMP philosophy despite the stilted prose. The handbook has current details for registering for the Match and describes the couples match and shared-residency positions. It also supplies concise explanations for rank-order lists and supplemental rank lists. However, some of the juiciest information is stored in the appendices, including selected statistics from the previous Match, NRMP policy statements, and an explanation of the Match algorithm. Finally, the handbook's back cover lists key dates for the Match process.

## NRMP Handbook for Independent Applicants

Like the *NRMP Handbook for Students*, this free publication from the NRMP is a must-read for independent applicants. You can get a copy by calling the NRMP at (202) 828-0566. The version for independent applicants covers the same topics as the general student handbook. In addition, the *Handbook for Independent Applicants* contains guidelines for verification of credentials for Match eligibility, a NRMP publication order form, and match dates for specialties covered in the NRMP's Specialties Matching Services (eg, dermatology).

## NRMP Directory/Hospitals and Programs Participating in the Matching Program

The *NRMP Directory* is a catalog of residency programs participating in the Match. Part I of the directory organizes the programs by hospital. Use this section to see what other specialty training programs are offered at the hospitals you're interested in. For example, since the presence of an internal medicine program typically means a lower caliber of training for family practice residents, family practice applicants may want to find hospitals without medicine programs. Part II lists programs by specialty type and is much more useful. You should receive the edition for the previous Match at no cost upon registration. You will also receive a revised edition for your Match late in the fall.

## NRMP Program Results/Listing of Filled and Unfilled Programs for the Match

If you want to find out which programs in your specialty were not filled last year, then this is the book to get. It's like going through someone's dirty laundry. The *NRMP Program Results* is given to unmatched applicants on Unmatch Day, who subsequently must enter the Scramble. Part II lists programs that did not fill all their spots. It can be a real eye-opener and give you a better feel for regional trends in competitiveness. If you are a marginal candidate applying in a competitive specialty, you may consider applying to several of the programs that went unfilled last year. But be forewarned—they probably went unfilled for good reasons. Though this publication is supposedly free only for applicants who failed to find placements in the previous Match, check your school's student affairs office for a copy.

## A⁺ NRMP Data

This must-have publication contains exhaustive data on the previous year's Match. It tracks Match trends over several years and puts you and your target specialty into perspective. Many of the tables are informative, but you'll want to check out a few choice ones (Table 1–4). Most students erroneously believe that the Match data are confidential. They aren't, if you can come up with $7 plus shipping, or if you choose to consult the copy in your school's student affairs office. Unfortunately, many student affairs offices operate on the belief that this data is confidential or that students don't really need these details.

## B Universal Application for Residency and Program Designation Card

You get one or two Universal Applications free when you sign up for the Match. There should be no need to purchase additional copies. Because you send a photocopy of the Universal Application to the few programs that accept it, simply photocopy your application if you need more copies (ie, as a worksheet). For detailed advice on completing the Universal Application, see Chapter 5.

## B Program Designation and Acknowledgment Card

This self-addressed card to acknowledge receipt of your application is a bit lame; it has no space for the program secretary to acknowledge receipt of other materials for your dossier, such as letters of recommendation and medical school transcripts. You can easily design a more useful acknowledgment card yourself (see "Application Complete Postcard," pg. 102). One free card comes with your Universal Application.

| TABLE 1–4. Must-see tables/charts. | |
|---|---|
| **Tables/Charts** | **What to Look For** |
| Applicants in the Matching program | Detailed Match statistics, grouped by applicant category. Compares U.S. seniors to foreign graduates. |
| PGY-1 positions, active applicants, and Match rates | Presents similar information as previous table, but in the context of the number of PGY-1 positions available. |
| Positions offered and % filled by U.S. seniors and total applicants | Breaks down Match fill rates over the previous 5 years by specialty. Allows you to spot trends in each specialty. |
| Programs, positions, ranked and filled | The rank/position value is the average number of times each position offered by that specialty was ranked. A rank/position value roughly corresponds to the degree of competitiveness—the higher the number, the tougher it is to get the spot. |
| U.S. seniors unmatched | Highlights the specialties in which students have had the most difficulty matching. |

# REFERENCES

Graettinger JS, Peranson E: The matching program. *N Engl J Med* 1981;304:1163.

Medschool.com website (http://www.medschool.com)

National Residency Matching Program, *Handbook for U.S. Medical Students, 2000 Match*. Washington, DC, 1999.

National Residency Matching Program, *Advanced Copy of Results and Data, 2000 Match*. Washington, DC, 2000.

National Residency Matching Program, 1999 *NRMP Data: 1999*. Washington, DC, 1999.

National Residency Matching Program, 1998 *NRMP Data: 1998*. Washington, DC, 1998.

National Residency Matching Program, 1997 *NRMP Data: 1997*. Washington, DC, 1997.

National Residency Matching Program, 1996 *NRMP Data: 1996*. Washington, DC, 1996.

# Setting Up the Fourth Year

## HOW DO I PICK AN ADVISER?

During your first 3 years of medical school, you may have identified or been assigned an academic adviser who shepherded you through a variety of situations, from surviving gross anatomy to helping you choose a medical specialty. If your adviser is an internist and you want to go into internal medicine, you may already be in great shape. However, if you choose a field different from that of your adviser or if your adviser does not closely monitor your application and matching process, then you need someone else to provide you with additional advice.

In selecting an adviser, you want someone who is savvy about a wide variety of factors regarding your career choice and the Match (Figure 2–1). Your adviser should be able to keep you informed of both academic and economic trends as well as training and job opportunities in your chosen field. They should be familiar with the strong and weak points of your candidacy, and they should know you well enough to offer personal, honest advice. Find an adviser who is familiar with the programs in which you are interested. For example, an adviser who trained on the East Coast may not be familiar with the West Coast programs. If you are interested in academic medicine, do not choose an adviser who is primarily involved in private practice (or vice versa). Your adviser should be able to answer a range of questions about the application process, from matters of fact (When are the deadlines?) to advice (Whom should I ask for recommendations?).

Some students advocate a dual-adviser system: one adviser to assist you with the "nuts and bolts" of the process and a more senior, well-known faculty member whose connections and telephone lobbying might open more doors for you.

How do you find such an adviser? Start by asking students in the class ahead of you about outstanding faculty members in your specific discipline. Your current medical school adviser may also have some suggestions. The dean of students often can guide you to the appropriate advisers. Ask the chairman of the department or the residency director at your school who they would recommend. The best advisers are junior or senior faculty who are involved in residency selection and who have advised applicants in previous years. When trying to identify the ideal adviser, be aware of the following potential pitfalls:

**ADVISERS SHOULD SERVE AS BOTH COUNSELOR AND ADVOCATE.**

**FIGURE 2-1**

☐ Discuss current academic and economic trends in the field
☐ Point out research opportunities
☐ Provide overall view of the application process
☐ Offer honest assessment of your competitive standing
☐ Highlight programs most appropriate for you
☐ Review and critique your application (eg, personal statement, CV)
☐ Conduct a mock interview
☐ Review your rank-order list
☐ Make key "political" phone calls if necessary
☐ Be available on Unmatch Day

Checklist for the career adviser.

- **Adviser overload:** A specific person counseling so many students that you're left with little attention (this can also be a problem with recommenders who write many letters each year).
- **Adviser oversight:** He or she tends to misjudge a student's competitiveness or the competitiveness of the field.
- **Adviser nostalgia:** A faculty member who remembers what it was like in your field many years ago, but no longer has an accurate perception of the Match.
- **Adviser bias:** One who gives all students the same "pet" list of programs to apply to regardless of their personal career goals, geographic constraints, or the strength of an applicant's candidacy.

## WHEN SHOULD I SCHEDULE MY ACTING INTERNSHIPS?

Figure 2–2 offers a checklist/time line for organizing Match activities during your fourth year in medical school. Conventional wisdom says that you should do at least one acting internship (AI; aka subinternship, externship, junior internship, or senior clerkship) in your target specialty early in your fourth year (or late in your third year at some schools). Your evaluation during this rotation is one of the most influential factors considered by the selection committee. In addition, a strong letter of recommendation from an attending physician on this rotation is usually critical to a competitive application. Some programs will expect at least one letter of recommendation from an AI (if you did one) as part of your application. Verify with the dean's office the last rotation block that will show up in your dean's letter and on your transcript (usually September).

Because of the importance of this rotation, many students like to do a "warm-up" rotation before going all out on the AI. For example, students interested in internal medicine often rotate on cardiology, infectious disease, or emergency medicine before an internal medicine AI. The warm-up rotation allows you to acquire the experience, knowledge, and skills (political and manual) that are necessary for success on your AI. The warm-up rotation also ensures that you enter the AI refreshed and enthusiastic. However, don't relax too much; strong grades or evaluations within electives of your target specialty are also highly regarded by the selection committee. Stu-

KEEP IN MIND THE LAST SENIOR BLOCK THAT WILL APPEAR IN YOUR DEAN'S LETTER.

SCHEDULE THE AI AFTER YOUR SUMMER BREAK OR A LIGHT "WARM-UP" ROTATION.

**FIGURE 2-2**

| Task | Page | Mar | Apr | May | June | July | Aug | Sep | Oct | Nov | Dec | Jan | Feb | Mar | Apr | May |
|---|---|---|---|---|---|---|---|---|---|---|---|---|---|---|---|---|
| ☑ Choose/meet with career adviser | 13 | ■ | ■ | ■ | ■ | | | | | | | | | | | |
| ☑ Plan senior year — subIs, electives, audition rotations, etc. | 14 | ■ | ■ | ■ | | | | | | | | | | | | |
| ☑ Enroll in Match | 73 | | ■ | ■ | ■ | | | | | | | | | | | |
| ☑ Request program applications | 78 | | | ■ | ■ | ■ | | | | | | | | | | |
| ☑ Request letters of recommendation | 101 | | | ■ | ■ | ■ | | | | | | | | | | |
| ☑ Create CV | 105 | | | ■ | ■ | ■ | | | | | | | | | | |
| ☑ Create personal statement | 117 | | | ■ | ■ | ■ | | | | | | | | | | |
| ☑ Buy interview clothes | 164 | | | | | ■ | ■ | | | | | | | | | |
| ☑ Take application photos | 101 | | | | | ■ | ■ | | | | | | | | | |
| ☑ Review/request dean's letter and transcripts | 97 | | | | | | ■ | ■ | | | | | | | | |
| ☑ Mail application materials | 89 | | | | | | ■ | ■ | | | | | | | | |
| ☑ Schedule interviews/follow-up applications | 161 | | | | | | | ■ | ■ | ■ | | | | | | |
| ☐ Interview at programs | 181 | | | | | | | | ■ | ■ | ■ | | | | | |
| ☐ Write follow-up letters | 189 | | | | | | | | | ■ | ■ | ■ | | | | |
| ☐ Create/submit rank lists | 191 | | | | | | | | | | | | ■ | | | |
| ☑ Thank adviser and letter writers | 197 | | | | | | | | | | | | ■ | ■ | | |
| ☐ Send in *First Aid for the Match* surveys | 205 | | | | | | | | | | | | | ■ | | |
| ☐ Sign residency contract | 198 | | | | | | | | | | | | | | ■ | |

*Match Day!* (between Feb and Mar, at Thank adviser row)

First Aid for the NRMP Match time line.

dents interested in surgical specialties (eg, orthopedics, ENT, neurosurgery) often elect to do a general surgery AI before doing an AI in their specific interest in order to hone their floor management and operating room skills.

If you choose to do a second AI, either by requirement or by desire, note that there are good reasons for doing them early as well as for postponing them (Table 2–1).

| TABLE 2–1. Deciding when to do your second AI. |
|---|
| **Advantages of Doing Second AI Early** |
| • Offers another chance for a strong letter of recommendation (especially if third-year performance was weak)<br>• Strong evaluation on dean's letter a major plus<br>• Allows for a cushy spring schedule |
| **Advantages of Doing Second AI Late** |
| • Evaluation won't be included in dean's letter; more freedom to dictate learning objectives<br>• Tough rotations are distributed more evenly in fourth year; prevents burnout |

## WHEN SHOULD I SCHEDULE TIME FOR INTERVIEWS?

For the majority of students, interview dates run from November to early February. Students participating in "early Matches" (eg, ENT, neurosurgery, urology, ophthalmology) should leave time for interviews in November and early December. Most students take a month off for interviews, starting right before or after Christmas break. Unless you are considering a smaller number of programs in a limited geographic area, a 2-week Christmas break is usually not enough time.

Students who interview in January may have a slight advantage over those who interview earlier. Because their interviews occur after the holidays, committee members more readily remember the specifics of their applications and can push for them during highly charged ranking sessions. In addition, it may be hard for you to remember the specifics of a program you visited in December when making your rank list in February. If you interview early, consider revisiting programs that you plan to rank highly in order to refresh your memory and to reiterate your interest to the selection committee.

However, if you plan to hit many programs in the Northeast or upper Midwest, January may be a bad month because of winter traveling conditions. During the first week of January, one of us got stranded at a subway stop in a blizzard while visiting a program in Cleveland. A half-hour trip from the airport to the university turned into a two-and-a-half-hour ordeal. In January 1999, many students got caught in a Chicago blizzard for three days, and missed subsequent interviews. So allow extra time during snow season for visiting programs in these areas.

## SHOULD I STICK AROUND MY SCHOOL ON MATCH DAY?

The month featuring Match Day (March for most applicants) is generally not a good time to be vacationing or doing electives outside the country. If you feel the need to flee, choose another time. A certain percentage of U.S. medical students and international medical graduates will not be placed on Match Day and will have to enter the Scramble. If you do not match and have to enter the Scramble or if there is a problem with your rank list, you'll need to be in close communication with your dean and your adviser, either in person or by phone. This is especially true if you are trying to match in a

**PLAY IT SAFE. BE IN THE COUNTRY AROUND MATCH DAY.**

competitive specialty. If you must be out of the country, make contingency plans with your dean and adviser, and find access to a fax machine. The WEBROLIC system will allow you to find out if and where you matched via the Internet but keep in mind that many students will be logging in on Match Day and it may be easier to call your dean's office.

## SHOULD I DO AUDITION ROTATIONS?

Early in the fourth year, many students do audition rotations (away rotations or externships) at other schools in their target specialties to find out more about a specific program or to improve their chances of entering that program. Be careful. An away rotation is a two-edged sword—you can stumble as well as shine. Remember that you will probably be compared with medical students at that institution who are already familiar with the hospital environment and its faculty.

On the positive side, many programs will grant visiting students a "courtesy interview" at the end of an audition rotation. In fact, some programs in certain very competitive specialties, such as orthopedic surgery or emergency medicine, only take "known quantities"—students who have done rotations on site.

For the rest of you, consider doing away rotations only if you are aiming for a long-shot program in which you would not otherwise have a chance. If people from your medical school have matched at the program that you are considering, keep in mind that the program likely has a positive impression of your medical school and an away rotation may diminish your candidacy. If no one from your school has ever matched at that program, an audition rotation may give you that "foot in the door" as long as you do an excellent job. In evaluating the potential benefits of an audition rotation, you must size up whether you come across better in person or on paper. If you simply want to find out more about a program at a specific institution, consider doing an away rotation there but not in your target specialty (eg, emergency medicine at an institution whose surgery program interests you). Otherwise, you risk exposing yourself to unnecessary scrutiny.

## WHAT ABOUT OTHER ELECTIVES?

Your fourth year is a fantastic opportunity to fulfill your intellectual and personal curiosity by sampling all that medicine has to offer. Don't waste it! Though it's wise to take an elective or two that will prepare you for internship (Table 2–2), do not try to duplicate your internship during your fourth year: You'll get more than enough experience during your residency training. In addition, you might enjoy taking some electives that might not be available to you ever again. Your career adviser should have some good suggestions for fourth-year electives, as will students in the class ahead of you.

## WHEN SHOULD I SCHEDULE VACATION?

Don't forget to take time for yourself. Some students take a light rotation during September of their fourth year or take 2 weeks off during that period so that they can take care of residency applications. Remember that once residency starts, you will be limited to 2 to 5 weeks of vacation per year—

AUDITION ROTATIONS CAN HURT AS MUCH AS THEY HELP.

FULFILL YOUR LEARNING DESIRES WITHOUT DUPLICATING YOUR INTERNSHIP.

**TABLE 2–2. Recommended fourth-year electives by specialty.**

| Specialty | Recommended Electives for Internship | Related Electives |
|---|---|---|
| Anesthesiology | Surgical ICU | Radiology, emergency medicine, medical ethics |
| Dermatology | Infectious disease, medicine subinternship, pathology | Emergency medicine, ophthalmology, pediatric subinternship |
| Emergency medicine | ICU, radiology, gynecology, trauma surgery | Cardiology, dermatology, psychiatry crisis center, toxicology |
| Family practice | Cardiology, emergency medicine, gastroenterology, orthopedics | Dermatology, ophthalmology, overseas elective, radiology, sports medicine |
| Internal medicine | Cardiology, emergency medicine, infectious disease, pulmonary | Dermatology, orthopedics, OB/GYN, otolaryngology, overseas elective |
| Neurology | Psychiatry subinternship, radiology, geriatrics | Neurosurgery, emergency medicine |
| Obstetrics & gynecology | Maternal/fetal medicine, pediatrics, surgery subinternship, urology | Emergency medicine, family practice, endocrinology |
| Orthopedics | Emergency medicine, trauma surgery | ICU, rheumatology, radiology, sports medicine |
| Otolaryngology | Emergency medicine, neurology, surgery subinternship | Dermatology, pulmonary medicine |
| Ophthalmology | Emergency medicine, neurology | Dermatology, medicine consult |
| Pathology | Clinical anatomy, radiology | Laboratory medicine, infectious disease, hematology |
| Pediatrics | Emergency medicine, dermatology, pediatric infectious disease, pediatric intensive care medicine | Child psychiatry, medicine consult, radiology, pediatric surgery |
| Psychiatry | Endocrinology, neurology subinternship, medicine consult | Emergency medicine, toxicology, substance abuse |
| Radiology | Clinical anatomy, anatomic pathology | Informatics, orthopedics, emergency medicine |
| Surgery | Emergency medicine, ICU, trauma surgery, clinical anatomy | Medicine consult, surgical pathology, anesthesiology |

and you can probably forget holidays such as Christmas, Hanukkah, and Thanksgiving.

Consider spending part of your vacation at a major national meeting in one or two of your top specialty choices late in your third year or early in your fourth year, especially if the meeting is nearby or if your adviser is planning to go. A list of national meetings is published regularly in the *Journal of the American Medical Association*, on specialty organization websites (Table 2–3), as well as in the "Specialty Profiles" section of the Medschool.com website (http://www.medschool.com). Most of these conferences have special reduced

**ATTEND A MAJOR NATIONAL MEETING IN YOUR DESIRED SPECIALTY.**

**TABLE 2–3. Partial list of specialty organizations.**

| Specialty | Organization/Contact Information | Website |
|---|---|---|
| General | American Medical Women's Association (AMWA)<br>801 N. Fairfax Street, Suite 400<br>Alexandria, VA 22314<br>(703) 838-0500<br>Fax: (703) 549-3864 | http://amwa-doc.org |
| | American Medical Association (AMA)<br>515 North State Street<br>Chicago, IL 60610<br>(312) 464-5000 | http://www.ama-assn.org |
| | American Medical Student Association (AMSA)<br>1902 Association Drive<br>Reston, VA 20191<br>(703) 620-6600<br>Fax: (703) 620-5873 | http://www.amsa.org |
| Anesthesiology | American Society of Anesthesiologists (ASA)<br>520 North Northwest Highway<br>Park Ridge, IL 60068<br>(708) 825-5586 | http://www.asahq.org |
| Dermatology | American Academy of Dermatology (AAD)<br>930 North Meacham Road<br>Schaumburg, IL 60173-4965<br>Phone: (708) 330-0230, ext. 365,<br>(888) 462-DERM | http://www.aad.org |
| Emergency medicine | American College of Emergency Physicians (ACEP)<br>P.O. Box 619911<br>Dallas, TX 75261-9911<br>(214) 550-0911,<br>(800) 798-1822 | http://www.acep.org |
| | Society for Academic Emergency Medicine (SAEM)<br>901 N. Washington Avenue<br>Lansing, MI 48906-5137<br>(517) 485-5484 | http://www.saem.org |
| | American Academy of Emergency Medicine (AAEM)<br>611 East Wells Street<br>Milwaukee, WI 53202<br>(800) 884-2236 | http://www.aaem.org |
| | Emergency Medicine Residents Association (EMRA)<br>P.O. Box 619911<br>Dallas, TX 75261-9911<br>(972) 550-0920 or (800) 798-1822<br>Fax: (972) 580-2829 or (972) 580-2816 | http://www.emra.org |
| Family practice | American Academy of Family Physicians (AAFP)<br>11400 Tomahawk Creek Parkway<br>Leawood, KS 66211-2672<br>(800) 274-2237 ext. 5224 or<br>(913) 906-6000 ext. 5224 | http://www.aafp.org |
| Internal medicine | American College of Physicians (ACP)<br>Independence Mall West Sixth Street<br>Philadelphia, PA 19106-1572<br>(800) 523-1546 | http://www.acponline.org |
| | American College of Preventive Medicine (ACPM)<br>1600 L Street NW<br>Suite 206<br>Washington, DC 20036<br>(202) 466-2044 | http://www.acpm.org |
| | American Geriatric Society (AGS)<br>770 Lexington Avenue<br>Suite 300<br>New York, NY 10021<br>(212) 308-1414 | http://www.americangeriatrics.org |

**TABLE 2–3. Partial list of specialty organizations. (continued)**

| Specialty | Organization/Contact Information | Website |
|---|---|---|
| Neurology | American Academy of Neurology (AAN)<br>2221 University Ave, Southeast, #335<br>Minneapolis, MN 55414<br>(612) 623-2400 | http://www.aan.com |
| Neurosurgery | American Association of Neurological Surgeons (AANS)<br>22 S. Washington<br>Parkridge, IL 60068<br>(847) 692-9500 | http://www.aans.org |
| Obstetrics and Gynecology | American College of Obstetricians and Gynecologists (ACOG)<br>409 12th Street SW<br>Washington, DC 20024<br>(202) 638-5577 | http://www.acog.org |
| Ophthalmology | American Academy of Ophthalmology (AAO)<br>P.O. Box 7424<br>San Francisco, CA 94120-8500<br>(415) 561-8500 | http://www.eyenet.org |
| Orthopedics | American Academy of Orthopedic Surgeons (AAOS)<br>6300 North River Road<br>Rosemont, IL 60018-4262<br>(708) 823-7186 | http://www.aaos.org |
| Otolaryngology | American Academy of Otolaryngology—<br>Head and Neck Surgery<br>1 Prince Street<br>Alexandria, VA 22314<br>(703) 836-4444 | http://www.entnet.org |
| Pathology | College of American Pathologists (CAP)<br>325 Waukegan Road<br>North Field, IL 60093<br>(800) 323-4040 | http://www.cap.org |
| | American Society of Clinical Pathologists (ASCP)<br>2100 West Harrison Street<br>Chicago, IL 60612-3798<br>(312) 738-1336 | http://www.ascp.org |
| Pediatrics | American Academy of Pediatrics<br>141 Northwest Point Blvd<br>Elk Grove Village, IL 60007<br>(800) 433-9016, ext. 7914 or<br>(708) 228-5005, ext. 7914 | http://www.aap.org |
| Physical Medicine and Rehabilitation | American Academy of Physical Medicine and Rehabilitation (AAPM&R)<br>One IBM Plaza, Suite 2500<br>Chicago, IL 60611-3604<br>(312) 464-9700<br>Fax: (312) 464-0227 | http://www.aapmr.org |
| Psychiatry | American Psychiatric Association (APA)<br>1400 K Street NW<br>Washington, DC 20005<br>(202) 682-6000 | http://www.psych.org |
| | American Academy of Child Psychiatry (AACAP)<br>3615 Wisconsin Avenue NW<br>Washington, DC 20016<br>(202) 966-7300 | http://www.aacap.org |
| Radiology | American College of Radiology (ACR)<br>1891 Preston White Drive<br>Reston, VA 22091<br>(800) ACR-LINE, (703) 648-8900 | http://www.acr.org |

**TABLE 2–3. Partial list of specialty organizations. (continued)**

| Specialty | Organization/Contact Information | Website |
|---|---|---|
| Radiology | Radiology Society of North America (RSNA)<br>820 Jorie Boulevard<br>Oak Brook, IL 60523-2251<br>(630) 571-2670<br>Fax: (630) 571-7837 | http://www.rsna.org |
| Radiation Oncology | American College of Radiation Oncology (ACRO)<br>820 Jorie Boulevard<br>Oak Brook, IL 60523<br>(630) 368-3733<br>Fax: (630) 571-7837 | http://www.acro.org |
|  | American Society for Therapeutic Radiology and Oncology (ASTRO)<br>12500 Fair Lakes Circle<br>Suite 375<br>Fairfax, VA 22033-3882<br>(800) 962-7876, (703) 502-1550<br>Fax: (703) 502-7852 | http://www.astro.org |
| Surgery | American College of Surgeons<br>633 N. St. Clair Street<br>Chicago, IL 60611<br>(312) 202-5000 | http://www.facs.org |
|  | American College of Chest Physicians<br>3300 Dundee Road<br>Northbrook, IL 60062<br>(847) 498-1400 | http://www.chestnet.org |
|  | American College of Colon and Rectal Surgeons<br>85 West Algonquin Road, Suite 550<br>Arlington Heights, IL 60005<br>(847) 290-9184 | http://www.fascrs.org |
| Urology | American Urological Association (AUA)<br>Office of Education<br>2425 West Loop South<br>Suite 333<br>Houston, TX 77027-4207<br>(800) 282-7077<br>(713) 622-2700<br>Fax: (713) 622-2898 | http://www.auanet.org |

registration rates for medical students. Some students submit abstracts based on clinical cases, which may enable them to obtain travel and registration funding from the department and/or dean's office. Your career adviser can provide more detailed information about the best ones to attend. At these meetings, you can meet the field's celebrities, find out what's hot, hear about problems and politics, scope out the turf wars, etc. You can preview programs in the specialty by looking at research posters or by listening to scheduled faculty talks. Spending time at a major meeting will provide you with valuable insights and perspectives and can also make you a more knowledgeable and interesting candidate during interviews.

# REFERENCES

American Academy of Child Psychiatry (AACAP) website (http://www. aacap.org).
American Academy of Dermatology (AAD) website (http://www.aad.org).
American Academy of Emergency Medicine (AAEM) website (http://www.aaem.org).
American Academy of Family Physicians (AAFP) website (http://www.aafp.org).
American Academy of Neurology (AAN) website (http://www.aan.com).

American Academy of Ophthalmology (AAO) website (http://www.eyenet.org).

American Academy of Orthopedic Surgeons (AAOS) website (http://www.aaos.org).

American Academy of Otolaryngology—Head and Neck Surgery (http://www.entnet.org).

American Academy of Pediatrics (AAP) website (http://www.aap.org).

American Academy of Physical Medicine and Rehabilitation (AAPM&R) website (http:www.aapmr.org).

American Association of Neurological Surgeons (AANS) website (http://www.aans.org).

American College of Chest Physicians website (http://www.chestnet.org).

American College of Colon and Rectal Surgeons website (http://www.fascrs.org).

American College of Emergency Physicians (ACEP) website (http://www.acep.org).

American College of Obstetricians and Gynecologists (ACOG) website (http://www.acog.org).

American College of Physicians (ACP) website (http://www.acponline.org).

American College of Preventive Medicine (ACPM) website (http://www.acpm.org).

American College of Radiation Oncology (ACRO) website (http://www.acro.org).

American College of Radiology (ACR) website (http://www.acr.org).

American College of Surgeons website (http://www.facs.org).

American Geriatric Society (AGS) website (http://www.americangeriatrics.org).

American Medical Association (AMA) website (http://www.ama-assn.org).

American Medical Student Association (AMSA) website (http://www.amsa.org).

American Medical Women's Association website (http://www.amwa-doc.org).

American Psychiatric Association (APA) website (http://www.psych.org).

American Society for Therapeutic Radiology and Oncology (ASTRO) website (http://www.astro.org).

American Society of Anesthesiologists (ASA) website (http://www.asahq.org).

American Society of Clinical Pathologists (ASCP) website (http://www.ascp.org).

American Urological Association (AUA) website (http://www.auanet.org).

College of American Pathologists (CAP) website (http://www.cap.org).

Emergency Medicine Residents Association (EMRA) website (http://www.emra.org).

Fellowship and Residency Electronic Interactive Database Access (FREIDA) American Medical Association (AMA) (http://www.ama-assn.org/freida).

Medschool.com website (http://www.medschool.com).

National Resident Matching Program (NRMP) website (http://nrmp.aamc.org/nrmp).

Radiology Society of North America (RSNA) website (http://www.rsna.org).

Reference directories. JAMA 1995;273(21):1652.

Society for Academic Emergency Medicine (SAEM) website (http://www.saem.org).

Wagoner NE, Suriano R, Stoner JA: Factors used by program directors to select residents. *J Med Educ* 1986;61:10.

# Your Specialty and the Match

**3**

In Chapter 1, you were introduced to several different matches. It's not surprising that each match has its own set of rules and strategies for success. But even within the NRMP Match, each specialty calls for a different approach to preparing a successful application and interview. For example, psychiatry residency directors expect and appreciate in-depth personal statements with thorough exploration of an applicant's background and motives for entering the specialty. A surgery residency director, on the other hand, might toss the same statement out the window in disgust. In that director's opinion, personal statements ought to be as succinct as possible.

In this chapter, we briefly profile selected specialties (see Table 3–1 for factors considered by medical students in choosing a specialty). Some of the smaller specialties are not profiled here. We have organized the information and advice for each specialty under the following headings:

**Overview:** The specialty in terms of recent trends in the medical career market.

**Match Numbers:** An analysis of recent Match results.

**Application Tips:** Advice and guidance for the application process specific for that specialty.

**Interview Tips:** Advice and guidance for the interview visit specific to that specialty.

**For More Info . . . :** A collection of essential career and residency application resources for the specialty.

The **Overview,** a brief description of the specialty itself as well as a glance at its socioeconomic trends, summarizes student, resident, and faculty observations. It is **not** intended as a basis for the complex and critical process of specialty selection. For more in-depth information about the specialty, consult the following resources:

- ▶ Faculty and house staff in the field
- ▶ Brochures from the academic or certifying society in the field (listed under "For More Info . . .")
- ▶ Glaxo Wellcome Pathway Evaluation Program. This is a free half-day seminar sometimes offered by the dean's office that helps you match your interests to different specialties. These seminars feature the *Glaxo*

**DIFFERENT STROKES FOR DIFFERENT FOLKS.**

**TABLE 3–1. Most influential factors determining specialty choice.**

Type and range of patient problems encountered

Appropriateness for personality

Opportunity to make a difference in people's lives

Desire to help people

Intellectual appeal of the specialty

The challenge of diagnostic problems

Diversity of diagnosis and therapy

*Medical Specialties Survey* (1991), a catalog of medical specialties and subspecialties complete with descriptions, practitioner profiles, and anecdotal picks and pans. Contact your student affairs office for details.

▶ Taylor A: *How to Choose a Medical Specialty*, 2nd ed. Philadelphia: Saunders, 1993. This resource contains detailed descriptions of most medical specialties, together with work sheets and exercises that allow you to find specialties compatible with your interests.

# ANESTHESIOLOGY

Factors attracting students to careers in anesthesiology include brief but positive doctor/patient relationships, above-average income, immediate results, and a more flexible lifestyle than other specialties. Anesthesiologists play an integral part in the practice of medicine including the presurgical center, operating room, post-anesthesia care unit, intensive care unit, pain management center and throughout the hospital. The field offers significant respect, intellectual stimulation and a comfortable lifestyle. However, the field of anesthesiology gradually reached saturation in the mid 1990s, especially in major urban centers. Even outside big cities, many graduating anesthesiologists were reporting difficulty finding employment. However, at this point there was a sharp decline in residency applicants, resulting in a decline in new attendings. Currently there are more job opportunities for new attendings such that there are more applicants with better credentials attempting to enter the field resulting in increased competition. Opportunities for entering post-residency fellowship training in such areas as critical care, pain management, and respiratory care have also increased in recent years.

## Match Numbers

There were 802 total positions filled from the 1005 available, up from 657 positions filled last year (refer to Figure 3–1A). The rate of positions filled was 79.8% in 2000, having risen gradually from 45.6% in 1996 (Figure 3–1B). The percentage of positions filled by U.S. medical graduates has also risen gradually from a low 17.3% in 1996 to 54.5% in 2000 (Figure 3–1B). Although the number of positions offered by anesthesiology programs declined steadily from 1992 to 1996, they have continued to rise since then.

## Application Tips

With decreasing medical student interest in the specialty, the anesthesiology match is definitely a buyer's market. Most prestigious programs emphasize good clinical grades and strong letters of evaluation—especially from the anesthesiology attending physician or head of the anesthesiology depart-

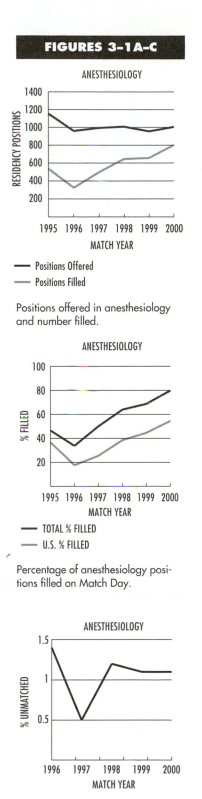

**FIGURES 3-1A–C**

ANESTHESIOLOGY

— Positions Offered
— Positions Filled

Positions offered in anesthesiology and number filled.

ANESTHESIOLOGY

— TOTAL % FILLED
— U.S. % FILLED

Percentage of anesthesiology positions filled on Match Day.

ANESTHESIOLOGY

Percentage of U.S. seniors unmatched in anesthesiology on Match Day.

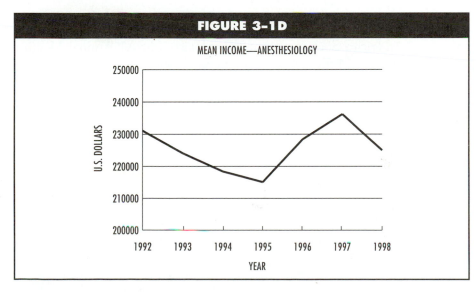

**FIGURE 3-1D**

MEAN INCOME—ANESTHESIOLOGY

Mean income of anesthesiologists in U.S. dollars.

ment—over board scores. Indeed, a recent study (based on data collected when anesthesiology was more competitive) demonstrated that only higher scores for letters of recommendation and interviews differentiated those that matched in anesthesiology from the applicant pool at large. All application material should be submitted by October. For the average to above-average student, advisers suggest that 10 to 15 applications are sufficient to get a comfortable 8 to 10 interviews. Plan to coordinate separate applications and interviews for internship positions. Often, hospitals can arrange interviews for internship and anesthesiology positions on the same day, so be sure to ask about this possibility when scheduling interviews.

## Interview Tips

Interviews are usually conducted in December and January. Typically, interview days begin at 8 AM and end early in the afternoon. Most interviews last 30 to 60 minutes, followed by a tour of the hospital and opportunities to speak with house staff. There are usually no difficult questions or pimping, but you may be asked your views of the specialty's future, including the decreasing job opportunities. Be prepared to discuss your ability to be a team player and work with other physicians, especially surgeons.

## For More Info . . .

▶ *American Society of Anesthesiologists Information Packet.* This free career information packet includes general articles (of marginal value) on the specialty itself, a directory of anesthesiology training programs as listed in the *Graduate Medical Education Directory*, and a directory of fellowships for specialized training in pain management. The packet can be obtained by contacting:

American Society of Anesthesiologists
520 North Northwest Highway
Park Ridge, IL 60068
(708) 825-5586
http://www.asahq.org

Global Anesthesiology Server Network (GASNet)
http://www.gasnet.org

National Meetings

American Society of Anesthesiologists (ASA) Annual Meeting
October 14 through 18, 2000 in San Francisco, CA.

## DERMATOLOGY

In general, established dermatologists enjoy good working hours, high income levels, a variety of procedures, and a typically healthy patient population. However, the field suffers from a poor distribution of physicians. There are openings available in smaller communities and rural areas, whereas most urban centers are saturated. With increasing emphasis on primary care, practicing dermatologists face cutbacks in their range and amount of work. The relatively routine and milder skin diseases are increasingly being treated by primary care physicians. As a result, more attention is being paid to the diagnosis of oncologic diseases, surgical procedures, and cosmetic treatments not covered by managed care contracts.

Specialty training in dermatology requires one year of internship, followed by three years of residency. A preliminary medicine year is preferable, but any training involving clinical patient care, such as surgery or transitional medicine, is usually acceptable. Residency training will include diagnostic and therapeutic procedures, both medical and surgical, with emphasis varying according to the particular program.

## Match Numbers

Dermatology continues to be one of the most difficult specialties to match. In 2000, 24.3% of U.S. seniors who applied in dermatology failed to match, up from 17.3% the year before (Figure 3–2C). In the same time period dermatology programs have continued to slightly increase the number of positions they offer, up from 241 positions in 1997 to 251 positions offered in 2000 (Figure 3–2A). Dermatology continues to be one of the most competitive specialties, with 100% of positions filled each year, 80.4% of which were U.S. medical students in 2000 (Figure 3–2B).

## Application Tips

Given the competitive nature of dermatology, all aspects of the residency application are important. Dermatology programs screen applicants intensively before offering interviews to prospective residents. Many use AΩA status, at least three honors in clinical rotations, high board scores, and a top-notch dean's letter as preliminary considerations. Competitive programs often use the USMLE Step 1 score to screen applications and research in dermatology is highly recommended. A glowing evaluation in the dermatology subinternship and supportive letters of recommendation are vital. However, given the competitive nature of the specialty, applicants need to demonstrate more than just academic excellence.

## Interview Tips

Since there are many stellar applicants in this small field, the interview is often a heavily weighted factor for acceptance. Dermatology programs usually offer interviews to about only 10 to 15% of their applicants. They may offer three to six interviews per day, lasting 30 to 45 minutes each. Depending on the program, interviews may be conducted by individual faculty members or by a panel consisting of three or more interviewers. Interviews are designed to measure the applicant's interest in the specialty and to evaluate his or her potential for contribution in the future, as well as to find out whether he or she would get along with other people in the department. The applicant is

**FIGURES 3–2A–B**

Positions offered in dermatology and number filled.

Percentage of dermatology positions filled on Match Day.

**A TRACK RECORD IN DERMATOLOGY RESEARCH IS CONSIDERED A BIG PLUS.**

FIGURE 3-2C

Percentage of U.S. seniors unmatched in dermatology on Match Day.

rarely pimped, but will be expected to discuss any prior research or involvement in dermatology intelligently and in detail.

## For More Info . . .

▶ *American Academy of Dermatology Information Packet.* This free information packet includes a mind-numbing description of accredited dermatology training programs and a list of dermatology programs worldwide as well as of dermatology fellowships in North America. The packet can be obtained by contacting:

American Academy of Dermatology
930 North Meacham Road
Schaumberg, IL 60173-4965
(708) 330-0230, ext 365
(888) 462-DERM
http://www.aad.org

National Meetings

Academy 2000: Meeting of the American Academy of Dermatology August 2 through 6, 2000 in Nashville, TN.

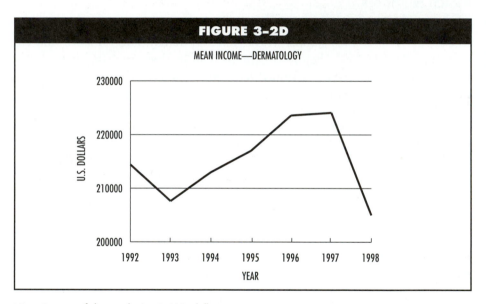

Mean income of dermatologists in U.S. dollars.

# EMERGENCY MEDICINE

Emergency medicine (EM) has enjoyed tremendous growth over the past few years, with good reason. Regular working hours, relatively abundant free time, and the ability to integrate medicine with surgical procedures all add to this field's appeal. This is also one of the few specialties in which one can become an attending straight out of residency training. Moreover, post-residency fellowships are plentiful and easily obtained for those desiring further training. EM physicians enjoy versatility and flexibility in pursuing such exotic fields as international health, disaster/rescue medicine, and diving medicine. And now with the television show "ER," it's a glamorous specialty to boot. Unfortunately, EM is infamous for a high burnout rate, attributable to high-stress working conditions, hostile patients, and the possibility of never-ending night shifts for junior attendings.

Residency programs in emergency medicine require either three or four years total training. In either case, the internship year is usually integrated with the main EM training. For the non-integrated programs, a separate internship year can be done in the field of medicine, surgery, or transitional medicine. The bulk of EM training time is spent in emergency rooms, learning resuscitation techniques, and treating both medical and trauma-related illnesses. However, residents will also rotate through specialties such as medicine, pediatrics, OB/GYN, surgery, anesthesiology, and orthopedic surgery to acquire a well-rounded knowledge and to develop an eye for common emergencies in these fields.

## Match Numbers

Competition for spots in emergency medicine residencies continues to intensify, despite the addition of positions to the 2000 match. In 2000, 1110 of the 1118 positions offered were filled (99.3% fill rate).(Figures 3–3A, 3–3B). This high fill rate marks an upward trend in the number of applicants to the field, as EM residencies become increasingly competitive. In fact, 6.6% of all U.S. seniors who applied in emergency medicine failed to match and had to scramble, up from 3.9% in 1999 (Figure 3–3C).

## Application Tips

Given the competitive nature of EM, all aspects of the residency application are important. It is especially critical to do well in an EM rotation and to ask for strong letters of recommendation from the attending physicians or the chief of emergency medicine. Letters from surgery, medicine, pediatrics, or OB/GYN are also well regarded. Competitive programs often use the USMLE Step 1 score to screen applications. To improve your chances with a very competitive program, consider doing an externship at that institution, especially if you are not particularly strong on paper (if you do the externship, prepare to excel). All application and supporting material, except for the dean's letter, should be submitted by early October. The optimal number of applications to submit depends on the candidate's strength, but many suggest 25 to 30 applications to yield 10 to 15 interviews.

## Interview Tips

Expect three to four interview sessions, typically lasting 30 to 60 minutes in length and conducted by the residency directors, attendings, and residents, as well as ER nurses and technicians. In general, interviewers are relaxed,

## FIGURES 3–3A–B

EMERGENCY MEDICINE

— POSITIONS OFFERED

— POSITIONS FILLED

Positions offered in emergency medicine and number filled.

EMERGENCY MEDICINE

— TOTAL % FILLED

— U.S. % FILLED

Percentage of emergency medicine positions filled on Match Day.

FIGURE 3-3C

Percentage of U.S. seniors unmatched in emergency medicine on Match Day.

friendly, and genuinely interested both in giving information about the programs and learning more about the applicant's personality.

## For More Info . . .

▶ *ACEP Student Information Packet*. The packet includes a directory of emergency medicine training programs. To obtain a copy, write or call:

American College of Emergency Physicians
P.O. Box 619911
Dallas, TX 75261-9911
(214) 550-0911
(800) 798-1822
http://www.acep.org

▶ Emergency Medicine Residents' Association (EMRA). In addition to the general information packet, you may wish to take out a student membership in the EMRA. A $45 annual fee provides you with a subscription to *Annals of Emergency Medicine*; *ACEP News*, a monthly newsletter; *EM Resident*, a bimonthly newsletter; and access to specialty meetings and conferences. Since the medical student affiliate (MSA) branch of EMRA was created in 1992, most information remains geared toward residents. To enroll, call:

Emergency Medicine Residents' Association
(800) 798-1822
http://www.emra.org

Society for Academic Emergency Medicine (SAEM)
901 Washington Avenue
Lansing, MI 48906-5137
(517) 485-5484
http://www.saem.org

American Academy of Emergency Medicine (AAEM)
611 East Wells Street
Milwaukee, WI 53202
(800) 884-2236
http://www.aaem.org

National Meetings

SAEM Annual Meeting
May 21 through 24, 2000 in San Francisco, CA
ACEP Scientific Assembly
October 23 through 26, 2000 in Philadelphia, PA
AAEM 7th Annual Scientific Assembly
February 22 through 25, 2001 in Orlando, FL at the Disney
    Coronado Springs Resort

For further reading:

▶ Delbridge, TR. *Emergency Medicine In Focus: A Handbook for Medical Students and Prospective Residents*. A compact guide to the emergency medicine residency application process. It is available to EMRA/ MSA members for $15. To order, call:

    ACEP Publications
    (800) 798-1822, touch 6

▶ Koscove, EM: An applicant's evaluation of an emergency medicine internship and residency. *Ann Emerg Med* 1990;19:774. This article offers an exhaustive collection of factors to consider when applying and interviewing at emergency medicine training programs.

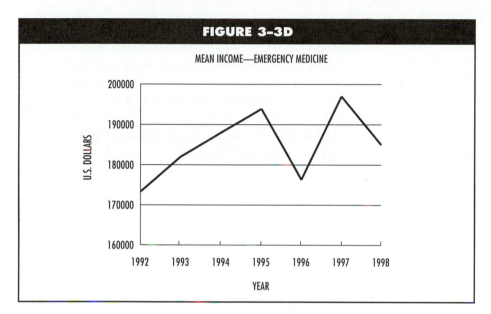

**FIGURE 3-3D**

MEAN INCOME—EMERGENCY MEDICINE

Mean income of emergency medicine physicians in U.S. dollars.

FAMILY PRACTICE

Positions offered in family practice and number filled.

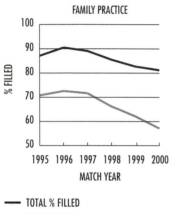

FAMILY PRACTICE

Percentage of family practice positions filled on Match Day.

> "EACH YEAR WE SEE APPLICANTS WHO ARE UNABLE TO REALLY TELL US WHY THEY WANT TO GO INTO FAMILY PRACTICE BECAUSE THEY DIDN'T HAVE ADEQUATE EXPERIENCE IN THE FIELD."
> — FAMILY PRACTICE RESIDENCY DIRECTOR

# FAMILY PRACTICE

Family practice (aka family medicine or family and community medicine) embraces the biopsychosocial model in its treatment of individuals and of the family as a whole. Students entering family practice have a strong commitment to primary care and enjoy the wide variety of patients and clinical problems encountered in this specialty, which spans medicine, pediatrics, OB/GYN, and surgery. Do not make the *faux pas* of calling this specialty *general practice*, as this term refers to the general practitioner (GP) of old who practiced general medicine immediately after internship. In today's world, an inexperienced GP can wave goodbye to good jobs in competitive locations.

Family practice graduates who are willing to practice medicine outside academic settings enjoy bright job prospects throughout the country, thanks especially to the growing presence of managed care. In an academic center, the family practice graduate can be an attending physician right out of residency. Though subspecialty opportunities are limited, sports medicine, geriatrics, and adolescent medicine are booming growth areas and very popular among residents. Finally, there is growing opportunity for fellowship training in academic subjects, which, for family practice, often focuses on epidemiology and public health.

In family practice, there is no consensus about the "best" programs. You can identify only the most "popular" programs, which depend on geographic region—university versus community versus rural. Note that curricula vary with geography, especially in the amount of obstetrics taught. The most formal training and education are afforded by a university setting; however, family practice here often gets trampled by internal medicine. Community-based programs usually have the run of the hospital; however, specialty training and didactic teaching often suffer. Rural-based programs are not as numerous as the others. Residents usually learn practical clinical skills and low-tech medicine in a non-academic, preceptorship-like atmosphere. The Midwest and the West Coast generally have a more favorable orientation toward family practice.

If your school does not have a family practice department, you will probably have to hustle to put together a strong application. Possible obstacles: lack of solid career guidance and no clinical experience to buttress your reasons for going into family practice. Plan to take extra steps to arrange a family practice preceptorship.

## Match Numbers

In 1996, a record 16.1% of U.S. seniors went into family practice, allowing the specialty to fill over 90.5% of its available positions (Figure 3–4B). However, the popularity of family practice seems to be decreasing, with the number of positions filled decreasing steadily from a high of 90.5% in 1996 to 81.2% in 2000. Nevertheless, 15.5% of applicants went into family practice, making it the second most popular specialty, after internal medicine, which received 23.4% total applicants. Only 1.7% of family practice applicants did not match in 2000, making it one of the easier specialties to match into (Figure 3–4C). Nearly one third of family practice positions available were filled by international medical graduates.

## Application Tips

Given the rising interest in family practice, some applicants are now finding that matching up with a good program is no longer a sure thing. In applying, keep the following considerations in mind. Programs want to see a strong commitment to family medicine. They favor experience in public health, as well as evidence of a mature, well-rounded personality. In addition, programs are more sensitive to your reasons for choosing family practice over internal medicine (especially primary care internal medicine). Program directors like to see a demonstrated interest in OB/GYN and pediatrics. Given the varying foci of different programs, you may consider customizing your personal statement to best address the training philosophies of each program or at least each type of program (university vs community vs rural). Like other primary care specialties, family practice residencies will scrutinize your personal statement very carefully. Indeed, aside from the interview, family practice residency directors in a recent study singled out the dean's letter, the personal statement, and transcripts as the most useful selection criteria.

Mail your applications no later than mid-October. Many programs actually grant interviews on a first-come, first-served basis. Submit as many applications as you wish. Students recommend interviewing at a minimum of six programs, with eight to ten being a more comfortable range.

## Interview Tips

Because family practice programs tend to be smaller, the visit (generally with two to four interviews) tends toward the personal. Prepare for "touchy-feely" type questions. Are you concerned with the human side of medicine? What do you want to do with your training in family practice? Work overseas for a few years? Do rural medicine? Focus on women's health? Think through these and similar questions. Reading up on social and ethical issues in medicine may help broaden your perspective and get you psyched for the interviews.

## For More Info . . .

▶ American Academy of Family Physicians
11400 Tomahawk Creek Parkway
Leawood, KS 66211-2672
(913) 906-6000

**FIGURE 3-4C**

FAMILY PRACTICE

Percentage of U.S. seniors unmatched in family practice on Match Day.

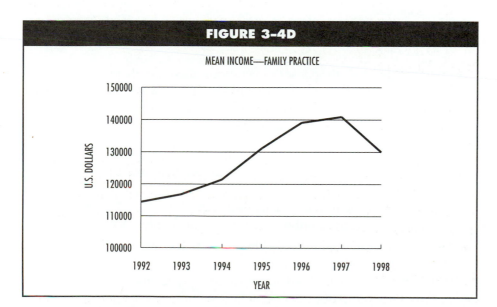

**FIGURE 3-4D**

MEAN INCOME—FAMILY PRACTICE

Mean income of family practice in U.S. dollars.

▶ **AAFP Student Membership**. For a mere $10 per year, you will receive a subscription to the journal *American Family Physician*, which features practical articles on family medicine topics; the newsweekly *AAFP Reporter*; and a directory of family practice clerkships/preceptorships for students desiring clinical experience in family practice. Membership is limited to medical students at LCME accredited medical schools. To enroll, contact:

> AAFP Membership Records
> (800) 274-2237

▶ **AAFP Publications.** The AAFP has a number of publications, many complimentary, aimed at medical students considering family practice:

> ▶ *Directory of Family Practice Residency Programs*. This is an annually revised database of family practice residencies, considered more accurate, more informative and more up-to-date than either FREIDA or the "Green Book." It is free to medical students through your school's family medicine department. Otherwise, the cost per copy is $10 for members, $15 for non-members.
>
> ▶ *Reprint 300*. This booklet contains definitions of family practice and family physicians; free on request.
>
> ▶ *Facts About Family Practice*. For number-crunchers, this book includes detailed statistics about family practice. Cost: $25 for members, $40 for non-members.
>
> ▶ *A Medical Student's Guide to Strolling Through the Match*—The what, when, where, why and how of residency selection.
>
> ▶ *Directory of Family Practice Clerkships/Preceptorships*
>
> ▶ *Residency Directory*—Information about more than 400 family practice residencies in the United States.
>
> ▶ *Residency Information Packet*—A packet designed for medical students seeking statistical and informative data on family practice residency programs. Additional information enclosed includes a listing of all ACGME-accredited family practice residency programs.

To order, call:

AAFP Order Department
(800) 274-2237

▶ Scherger JE et al: Responses to questions about family practice as a career. *Am Fam Physician* 1992;46(1):115. This article presents responses to 20 common questions about family practice; it is informative but reads like thinly veiled propaganda.

National Meetings

> National Conference of Family Practice Residents and Medical Students
> August 2–6, 2000 in Kansas City, Missouri
> (Students can register online at www.aafp.org/conference)
>
> American Academy of Family Physicians Scientific Assembly
> September 20–24, 2000 in Dallas, Texas
> Key Links: American Academy of Family Physicians
> http://www.aafp.org

# INTERNAL MEDICINE

Internal medicine programs are usually divided into "traditional" programs and primary care programs. Traditional medicine offers more of an inpatient focus, plus electives for sampling different subspecialties. Residents in primary care medicine have more of an outpatient experience and often receive additional training in gynecology and pediatrics. Students are often attracted to traditional internal medicine because it leaves the door open for further subspecialty training or generalist practice. On the other hand, students going into primary care internal medicine are often committed to primary care but are not as interested in the obstetrics, pediatrics and surgical assisting experience offered by family practice. Primary care internal medicine programs maintain that their graduates are better suited to enter community practice than are their traditional counterparts.

Many students are attracted to general internal medicine because of its emphasis on adult care, complex problem-solving, and continuity of care. Practical advantages include broadening job prospects for general internists, especially in managed care settings, and the flexibility to go into primary care or pursue subspecialty training. However, medicine subspecialists are currently facing an oversupply of subspecialists, bread and butter procedures lost to primary care physicians, and shrinking reimbursement schedules from Medicare and managed care plans.

## Match Numbers

Although the number of positions offered by internal medicine programs was at a record high of 4,810 in 2000, only 93.4% of those positions were filled, continuing the trend toward declining fill rates (Figures 3–5A and 3–5B). More than one third of the available internal medicine positions were filled by international medical graduates (Figure 3–5B).

## Application Tips

The best thing you can do for your internal medicine application is to pull down strong evaluations in your junior and senior medicine clerkships, as well as enthused letters of recommendations. Primary care programs place a bit more emphasis on the applicant's personal goals, skills, interests, and career plans in general internal medicine. Most competitive residency programs, including several of the most prestigious, couldn't care less about Step 1 scores as long as you passed. Externships are not the norm, unless you want to try to improve your chances at an otherwise long-shot program. Plan to submit all your residency applications and supporting material by the beginning of October; ignore those February application deadlines. Again, there are no hard and fast rules about the number of applications you should complete; however, some residency advisers suggest that the typical student send in 10 to 15 applications in order to secure interviews at 8 to 10 programs.

## Interview Tips

The typical interview day starts at 8 AM and goes to about 3 PM. Applicants usually receive two or three 20- or 30-minute interviews. In general, internal medicine programs conduct interviews in a relatively benign fashion; however, that does not mean that you can drop your guard. Be prepared for tough questions concerning personal strengths and weaknesses, medical ethics, or clinical scenarios.

Positions offered in internal medicine and number filled.

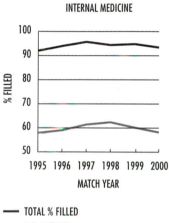

Percentage of internal medicine positions filled on Match Day.

Percentage of U.S. seniors unmatched in internal medicine on Match Day.

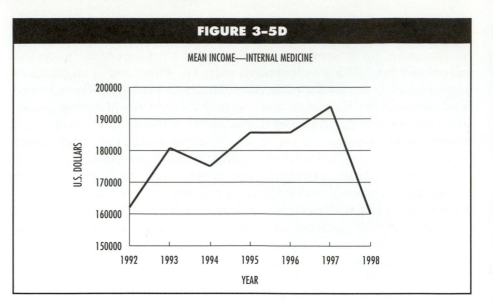

**FIGURE 3-5D**

MEAN INCOME—INTERNAL MEDICINE

Mean income of internists in U.S. dollars.

## For More Info . . .

▶ American College of Physicians (ACP)
Independence Mall West
Sixth Street at Race
Philadelphia, PA 19106-1572
(800) 523-1546
http://www.acponline.org

▶ American College of Preventive Medicine (ACPM)
1600 L. Street NW
Suite 206
Washington, DC 20036
Phone: (202) 466-2044
http://www.acpm.org

▶ American Geriatric Society (AGS)
770 Lexington Avenue
Suite 300
New York, NY 10021
Phone: (212) 308-1414
http://www.americangeriatrics.org

▶ American Gastroenterological Association (AGA)
7910 Woodmont Ave., 7th
Bethesda, MD 20814
Phone: (301) 654-2055
Fax: (301) 654-5920

National Meetings

The 2000 Annual Scientific Meeting of the American
Geriatrics Society
May 17 through 21, 2000 in Nashville, TN

# NEUROLOGY

Neurology has greatly benefited from the recent explosion in technological research. In the past few years, the specialty has grown and changed direction; the focus is now shifting towards treatment, traditionally its weak area. At this time, it is still unclear how the field will be affected by the current changes brought about by managed care systems. It is predicted that primary care physicians will take increasing responsibility for such chronic problems as stroke, headaches, and uncomplicated seizures. However, more complex neurological problems will still require the care of a specialist. Currently, job opportunities for neurologists seeking private practices are readily available. In fact, some studies project a major shortage (up to 30%) in the supply of neurologists by the year 2010. For those pursuing an academic career, however, recent cut-backs in NIH funding could make fellowship and research positions increasingly difficult to obtain.

Neurology requires a 3-year residency program preceded by an internship year in medicine, surgery, or transitional medicine. It generally works to the resident's advantage to choose a medicine internship, which tends to be more relevant to later training in neurology. Depending on the program, the training might focus on one or two areas, such as anatomic neurology, diagnosis, or treatment techniques. Also, keep in mind that the patient population may influence the quality and focus of training in certain areas (eg, trauma-related neurologic diseases, HIV disease, or such chronic problems as stroke and epilepsy).

## Match Numbers

The number of positions offered by neurology programs has increased over the past several years. As a result, the overall fill rate was at an all time high of 89.3% in 2000 (Figure 3–6B). The total number of applicants to neurology programs dropped 6% this year, but U.S. senior applications increased by 26%. Although there continues to be a high number of international medical graduates applying to neurology, the trend of positions offered to international medical graduates outnumbering those of U.S. seniors has shifted in favor of the U.S. senior by almost two to one this year (Figure 3–6B). The number of international medical graduates matched dropped from 251 in 1997 to 163 this year, while the number of U.S. seniors matched rose from 195 in 1997 to 303 this year. Almost all unmatched applicants are international medical graduates. The neurology match at present is a "two-tier" match for PGY-2 positions in that PGY-2 positions that did not fill in the previous Match are offered alongside the PGY-2 positions scheduled to begin in a year and a half. The number of vacancies left after the first tier match has dropped from 156 in 1995 to 28 in this match, a clear sign of improving conditions for the neurology Match.

## Application Tips

Positions for neurology residencies are filled through an early match, which requires applicants to be diligent in completing their applications as soon as possible. Although deadlines for most programs are in November or December, all information should be submitted by October. Senior neurology rotation(s) should be completed in the summer of the fourth year to ensure early letters of recommendation. This is one field where the reputation of the letter-writer counts as much as the letter's substance. Generally, you should ask for a letter from the best known and most senior members of the neurology

**FIGURES 3–6A–C**

Positions offered in neurology and number filled.

Percentage of neurology positions filled on Match Day.

Percentage of U.S. seniors unmatched in neurology on Match Day.

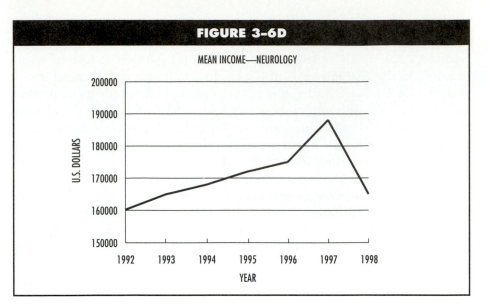

**FIGURE 3-6D**

MEAN INCOME—NEUROLOGY

Mean income of neurologists in U.S. dollars.

faculty, since their voices resonate loudest with the review committee. On another note, it could help to do away rotations at institutions of interest, although opinion is mixed on this issue.

To strengthen the application, include tangible proof of your commitment to the field of neurology, such as research experience, clinical volunteer experience, and publications. Some programs will also look at the location of your internship institution and the type of internship to which you applied. In general, many programs prefer a medical internship located at either the same institution or a similarly prestigious one.

## Interview Tips

Interviews range from individual sessions lasting about 30 to 45 minutes to group sessions conducted by a panel of faculty members. Each program has a different style, so be sure to ask about their format when you call to schedule the appointment. Most of the time, the questions posed will gauge your dedication to the field. In addition to the common interview fare (see Chapter 9), some interviewers ask applicants to describe their research projects or offer their opinions on ethical issues in neurologic diagnosis and treatment.

## For More Info . . .

▶ **Student information packet** available by calling or writing:

American Academy of Neurology
2221 University Ave, Southeast, #335
Minneapolis, MN 55414
(612) 623-2400
http://www.aan.com

▶ Other sources of information include:

American Board of Psychiatry and Neurology
500 Lake Cook Road, Suite 335
Deerfield, IL 60015-5249
Phone: (847) 945-7900
Fax: (847) 945-1146
http://www.abpn.com

San Francisco Matching Programs
P.O. Box 7584
San Francisco, CA 94120-7584
Phone: (415) 447-0350
Fax: (415) 561-8535
E-mail: help@sfmatch.org
http://www.sfmatch.org

# NEUROSURGERY

NEUROSURGERY

— POSITIONS OFFERED
— POSITIONS FILLED

Positions offered in neurosurgery and number filled.

NEUROSURGERY

— TOTAL % FILLED
— U.S. % FILLED

Percentage of neurosurgery positions filled on Match Day.

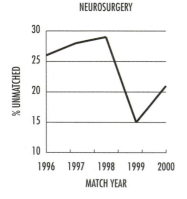

NEUROSURGERY

Percentage of U.S. seniors unmatched in neurosurgery on Match Day.

Neurosurgery is one of the most competitive fields in medicine. It is extremely rewarding, providing opportunities to participate in life saving procedures, and the ability to always learn something new and challenging. However, the specialty is notorious for long hours and irregular schedules and a high attrition rate. Neurosurgeons provide operative and non-operative management of lesions of the brain, spinal cord, peripheral nerves and their supporting structures. Neurosurgeons also participate in critical care and rehabilitation of paraplegia as well as other neurologic disorders, including the management of chronic pain conditions. This specialty requires manual dexterity and the ability to deal with both dramatic successes and failures. Neurosurgery is an extremely competitive specialty to apply to, with a consistently high unmatched rate each year. The need for neurosurgeons will be likely to increase secondary to new developments in autologous and fetal tissue transplantation and in stereotactic surgery for epilepsy.

Specialty training in neurosurgery requires one year in a general surgery internship, followed by five to six years of residency in neurosurgery. A minimum of 36 months of training must be spent in clinical neurosurgery and three months in clinical neurology. Residents may spend up to one year during their residency doing neurosurgery research.

## Match Numbers

Neurosurgery continues to be one of the most difficult specialties to match. The number of applicants has slowly declined since 1995. The fill rate of positions offered remains high, with 134 of 138, or 97.1% of positions offered being filled in 2000 (Figure 3–7A and 3–7B). Although the unmatch rate had decreased from 29% in 1998 to 15% in 1999, it rose again to 21% in 2000 (Figure 3–7C). The chances of international medical graduates matching in neurosurgery are poor, with approximately 75 to 90% of IMG applications not matching each year.

## Application Tips

Positions in neurosurgery are offered through the San Francisco Neurosurgery Matching Program. Given the intense competition in this specialty, applicants will fare better with a high USMLE Step 1 score (80th percentile or better), AΩA status, and honors in clinical rotations. Since neurosurgery is an early match specialty, the earlier the application is mailed the more chance of getting an interview. To improve your chances with a competitive program, consider doing an externship at that institution, especially if you are not strong on paper. All application and supporting material should be submitted by October. The average applicant submits 25 applications and interviews at nine programs. The optimal number of applications depends on your strength as a candidate, but it is recommended that you submit 30 to 40 applications and go to as many interviews as possible to increase your chances of matching.

## Interview Tips

Expect individual and/or group interviews lasting about 30 to 45 minutes.

## For More Info . . .

American Association of Neurological Surgeons (AANS)
22 S. Washington
Parkridge, IL 60068
Phone: (847) 692-9500
http://www.aans.org

American Board of Neurological Surgery
6550 Fannin Street, Suite 2139
Houston, TX 77030
(713) 790-6015
http://www.abns.org

San Francisco Neurosurgery Matching Program
PO Box 7584
San Francisco, CA 94120-7584
Phone: (415) 447-0350
Fax: (415) 561-8535
E-mail: help@sfmatch.org

National Meetings

Congress of Neurological Surgeons Annual Meeting
September 23 through 29, 2000, in San Antonio, TX

**FIGURES 3-8A-C**

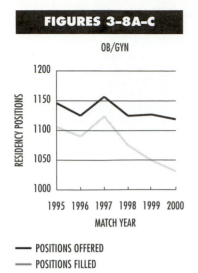

OB/GYN

— POSITIONS OFFERED
— POSITIONS FILLED

Positions offered in obstetrics and gynecology and number filled.

OB/GYN

— TOTAL % FILLED
— U.S. % FILLED

Percentage of obstetrics and gynecology positions filled on Match Day.

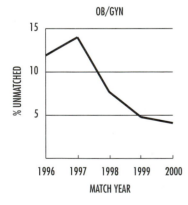

OB/GYN

Percentage of U.S. seniors unmatched in obstetrics and gynecology on Match Day.

# OBSTETRICS AND GYNECOLOGY

Obstetrics and gynecology has benefited from impressive biomedical advances in recent years. Improved maternal health care, *in vitro* fertilization, and better high-risk pregnancy management have expanded the practice of OB/GYN, allowing for better patient care. On the downside, the threat of litigation and the accompanying high professional liability insurance premiums continue to be key, thorny issues. Recent upgrading in the training of midwives and nurse practitioners to perform obstetrical duties further increases the competition for work within the field, prompting many OB/GYN practitioners to concentrate on gynecology.

In spite of the obstacles, demand to enter the field remains relatively strong. Medical students are attracted to the specialty because of the opportunity to work with a wide age range of women patients, the opportunity to provide long-term patient care, and the ability to combine basic medical care with surgical procedures.

Residencies in obstetrics and gynecology involve 4 years of training, followed by 2 years of post-graduate practice to become board-eligible. Patient care, including prenatal care, delivery techniques, routine gynecologic care, and gynecologic oncology care, make up the bulk of training. OB/GYN residents are eligible for certificates of specialty following 2- to 3-year post-residency fellowships in maternal-fetal medicine, gynecologic oncology, urogynecology, pelvic surgery, and reproductive endocrinology. On another note, keep in mind that programs at hospitals with religious affiliations may offer little or no experience in many aspects of infertility management, *in vitro* fertilization, and therapeutic and elective abortions.

## Match Numbers

Competition for training positions remains rigorous, especially on the West Coast. The falling number of deliveries and surgeries performed in teaching hospitals means that more programs in OB/GYN are cutting spots. In 2000, 1031 of the 1119 available residency spots were filled through the NRMP, a filling rate of 92.1% (Figures 3–8A and 3–8B). Meanwhile the number of spots filled by international medical graduates has risen steadily over the past five years, with 17% of positions filled by IMGs in 2000, up from 12.8% in 1999. The competitiveness of the specialty may be declining slightly, as the rate of applicants not matching was 4.1%, down from 4.8% the year before, and significantly decreased from 14% in 1997 (Figure 3–8C).

## Application Tips

It is important for interested applicants to complete a senior rotation in OB/GYN and to collect strong letters of support from well-known faculty members in this field. Some prestigious programs have suggested that students try to complete away rotations at institutions that interest them in order to increase their chances of being granted an interview. USMLE Step 1 scores, AΩA status, and the number of honors received are criteria used by many programs. Good evaluations in surgical rotations will also increase the applicant's strength. All application material should be submitted as early as possible, usually by October. The recommended number of applications depends on the strength of the applicant, but a general range of 15 to 20 is a fair norm to receive 10 to 15 interviews.

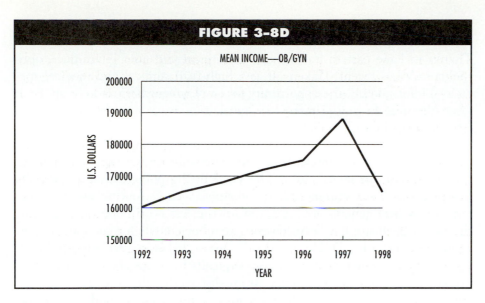

**FIGURE 3-8D**

MEAN INCOME—OB/GYN

Mean income of obstetricians and gynecologists in U.S. dollars.

For the 1996 Match, the AAMC introduced the Electronic Residency Application Service (ERAS) to OB/GYN as a replacement for the traditional "snail-mail" method of application. Most, if not all, OB/GYN programs now use ERAS for their sole method of application. Contact your dean's office or specific programs for details.

## Interview Tips

OB/GYN interviews are usually conducted in December and January. When you call to schedule, be aware that many programs have only a limited time period, during which they interview large groups of applicants. The earlier you submit your application, the more choices of dates you'll have. Interview schedules run long, lasting from 8 AM to 5 PM, with 3 to 4 interviews of 30 to 45 minutes each. These might be individual or group interviews, depending on the program. Be ready to present a case or to discuss some technical/ethical issues in the specialty. If you've done research, know your work inside-out, for you will be questioned on it. For the most part, interviews are cordial and informal, offering the interviewer an opportunity to assess your personality.

## For More Info . . .

▶ **Student information packet** available by calling or writing:

American College of Obstetricians and Gynecologists
409 12th Street, SW
Washington, DC 20024
(202) 638-5577

National Meetings

American Gynecological and Obstetrical Society (ACOG)
48th Annual Meeting
May 20 through 24, 2000, in San Francisco, CA

# OPHTHALMOLOGY

Thanks in large part to innovations in surgical and laser techniques, ophthalmology has recently taken off as a high-tech surgical and medical specialty. Unfortunately, the opportunity for employment has not kept up. As is often the case in non-primary care specialties, work in ophthalmology in large- and medium-sized cities is difficult to find, though not impossible. Because of the popularity of the training field, newly graduated ophthalmologists face sharpening competition with one another for the same patient pool, especially in larger cities. The cost-cutting policies that accompany managed care have shifted many procedures, such as routine vision check, refractions, and general eye care, toward the less costly optometrists. Furthermore, Medicare has been lowering reimbursements for cataract surgery. More patients with such chronic conditions as diabetes, glaucoma, and multiple sclerosis are being managed non-surgically by teams of optometrists and primary MDs. Some ophthalmologists are discovering that they have to market themselves to offer more than just surgical management of diseases in order to maintain a steady patient population.

Residencies in ophthalmology require a year of internship, followed by 3 years of specialty training. The residents often rotate through both surgical and non-surgical rotations, learning surgical techniques as well as medical diagnosis and management of eye diseases. Board eligibility is achieved immediately after finishing residency. Currently, there is no certification for subspecialties. However, residents can tailor their training to reflect areas of interest, such as cataract, glaucoma, or retinal surgery.

## Match Numbers

Ophthalmology remains one of the more competitive specialties. In the past several years, there has been a slow steady decline in the number of positions offered, while the number of applications has remained stable, resulting in an increasingly high filling rate of 98.8% in 2000 (Figure 3–9B). The non-match rate for U.S. seniors has risen from 6% in 1996 to 18% in 2000 (Figure 3–9C). International medical graduates continue to fare badly, with a non-match rate of 80% in 2000. In 2000, 429 of the 434 positions offered were filled, a 98.8% fill rate (Figures 3–9A and 3–9B).

## Application Tips

Positions in ophthalmology residencies are offered primarily through the Ophthalmology Matching Program conducted by August Colenbrander, MD. Given the competition to enter the field, the potential applicant should concentrate on doing well on the USMLE Step 1, in core senior electives, as well as the senior ophthalmology rotation. Supportive evaluations and recommendations from the senior ophthalmology faculty will clinch a strong application. Since this is another small field in which most department heads know one another, connections can play an important part in getting you that interview. Any research experience, especially work resulting in publications and/or presentations, should be included in your CV and will be viewed favorably. Most programs accept a universal application that must be submitted to a Central Application Service by mid-October. At present, most applicants are advised to submit about 20 to 35 applications. Many advisers also suggest that you apply to a mix of strong and weak programs in order to increase your probability of matching.

---

**UNDERSTAND THE DIFFERENCES BETWEEN OPHTHALMOLOGY AND OPTOMETRY, AND THEIR POLITICAL TURF BATTLES.**

**OPHTHALMOLOGY IS NOT AS COMPETITIVE AS IT USED TO BE.**

Positions offered in ophthalmology and number filled.

## Interview Tips

Similar to those of other surgical subspecialties, interviews for ophthalmology verge on the formal. Often, the applicants will meet with the department head, one or two senior faculty members, and at least one resident. Most interviews last from 30 to 45 minutes, with many of the questions geared toward assessing the applicant's interest in the field, clinical and research background, and personality. There could be some clinical questions asked, depending on the interviewer. Generally, take these interviews seriously, be professional and enthusiastic, but don't stress out. Interviewers do not ordinarily grill applicants. However, given the competitiveness of the field, interviewers sometimes ask about your contingency plans in case you don't match in ophthalmology.

## For More Info . . .

▶ *Envision Ophthalmology: A Practical Guide to Ophthalmology as a Career Choice.* A free publication of the American Academy of Ophthalmology, it includes general information about the application process, as well as a practical discussion of factors to consider in selecting and assessing an ophthalmology program. To receive this excellent career guide, call or write:

American Academy of Ophthalmology (AAO)
P.O. Box 7424
San Francisco, CA 94120-7424
(415) 561-8500
http://www.eyenet.org

▶ More information can be obtained from:

The American Board of Ophthalmology
111 Presidential Boulevard, Suite 241
Bala Cynwyd, Pennsylvania 19004-1075
Telephone: (610) 664-1175
Fax: (610) 664-6503
http://www.abop.org

**FIGURES 3-9B-C**

OPHTHALMOLOGY

— TOTAL % FILLED
— U.S. % FILLED

Percentage of ophthalmology positions filled on Match Day.

OPHTHALMOLOGY

Percentage of U.S. seniors unmatched in ophthalmology on Match Day.

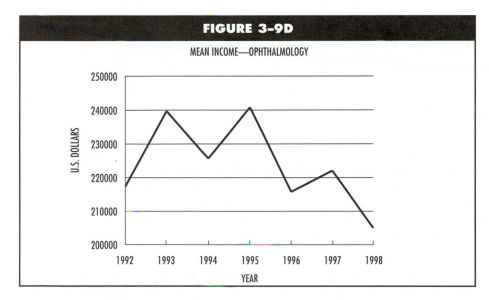

**FIGURE 3-9D**

MEAN INCOME—OPHTHALMOLOGY

Mean income of ophthalmologists in U.S. dollars.

Glaucoma Research Foundation (to inquire about research opportunities)
200 Pine Street, Suite 200
San Francisco, CA 94104
(415) 986-3162
(800) 826-6693
Fax: (415) 986-3763
http://www.glaucoma.org

San Francisco Match Ophthalmology Matching Program
PO Box 7584
San Francisco, CA 94120-7584
(For overnight delivery, send to 655 Beach Street, San Francisco, CA 94109)
Phone: (415) 447-0350
Fax: (415) 561-8535
E-mail: help@sfmatch.org
http://www.sfmatch.org

National Meetings

American Academy of Ophthalmology Annual Meeting
October 22 through 25, 2000, in Dallas, TX.

# ORTHOPEDICS

Orthopedic surgery continues to be a rewarding field. These specialists have opportunities to combine surgical techniques and orthopedic hardware (eg, microsurgery and joint prostheses) with work in physical rehabilitation for the treatment of acute and chronic orthopedic problems. Earnings for orthopedic surgeons continue to be well above average. However, increasing professional liability insurance premiums and overhead costs are reducing overall compensation.

Residencies require at least 5 years of training, with up to 2 years spent in general surgery or other approved medical or surgical residencies and the last 3 years in an orthopedic surgery program. A post-residency practice period is required before you become board-eligible. Subspecialty training is available in hand surgery, spinal surgery, sports medicine, orthopedic trauma, and pediatric orthopedics.

## Match Numbers

In 2000, 99.5% of the 554 available positions were filled through the Match, making orthopedic surgery among the most competitive surgical specialties. The number of positions offered by orthopedic surgery programs has risen consistently over the past several years, while the fill rate has remained stable at ~99% each year (Figures 3–10A and 3–10B). An increasing number of these positions are being filled by international medical graduates. The number of applicants not matching has decreased to 14.3% in 2000 from over 21% in 1999 (Figure 3–10C). Even so, orthopedics remains one of the highest non-match rates in the NRMP Match.

## Application Tips

Orthopedic surgery is becoming more academic. Thus, research experience is virtually a requirement for an application to be seriously considered by a prestigious program. Strong evaluations in the orthopedic surgery rotation, enthusiastic recommendations from the faculty members in the field, and high board scores are key ingredients of a strong application. It is common for residency programs to use USMLE Step 1 scores to screen applicants, with a cutoff ranging from the 75th to the 85th percentile. Some residency programs encourage students to take an audition elective at their institution in order to be considered for interviews. However, be aware that you will have to turn in a stellar performance on these away rotations. It would also help to select a mentor who has seniority in the department. Given the "good old boy" network at some institutions, establishing connections may open a few more doors. Deadlines for applications range from October to late December; however, be sure to send in all your application materials by early October, because interview spots fill quickly.

## Interview Tips

Interviews in orthopedic surgery are extremely difficult to obtain, so if you are offered one, it means that you've proven yourself academically. During the interviews, be prepared for anything. You could be asked questions probing personality type or to discuss a range of political, ethical, and sometimes, humorous subjects. Female applicants may encounter off-color remarks or inappropriate questions in a specialty that still sports a "jock" image. If you've done research, know your stuff so that you can answer questions quickly and

**ONE IN SEVEN U.S. SENIORS WENT UNMATCHED IN ORTHOPEDIC SURGERY.**

**HIGH BOARD SCORES, AΩA, MANY HONORS, AND RESEARCH ARE THE KEYS TO SUCCESS.**

### FIGURE 3-10A

ORTHOPEDICS

— POSITIONS OFFERED
— POSITIONS FILLED

Positions offered in orthopedics and number filled.

ORTHOPEDICS

— TOTAL % FILLED
⋯ U.S. % FILLED

Percentage of orthopedic positions filled on Match Day.

ORTHOPEDICS

Percentage of U.S. seniors unmatched in orthopedics on Match Day.

clearly. Interviewers mainly look for something distinctive about the person and try to determine whether he or she will fit in with the rest of the residents in the program. Interviews are usually conducted in middle to late November, December, January and early February. Interview days are quite long (6 to 8 hours) with four to five interviews. Interviews are mostly conducted on an individual basis, with three to four sessions of about 30 to 45 minutes each.

## For More Info . . .

► For a brochure on careers in orthopedic surgery, call or write:

American Academy of Orthopedic Surgeons
6300 North River Road
Rosemont, IL 60018-4262
(708) 823-7186
http://www.aaos.org

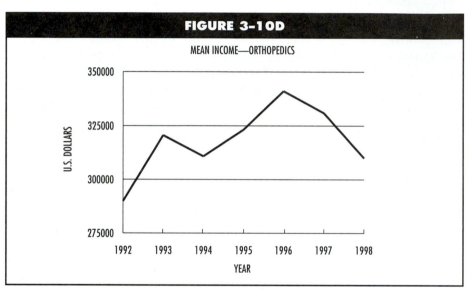

### FIGURE 3-10D

MEAN INCOME—ORTHOPEDICS

Mean income of orthopedic surgeons in U.S. dollars.

# OTOLARYNGOLOGY

Ear, nose, and throat (ENT) physicians will continue to be a small subspecialty in demand. Although the primary care specialties will likely take over allergy treatment and immunology as well as simple procedures like tympanotomy, ENT physicians will continue to have roles in academics, ENT oncology, and the growing fields of facial plastics and otologic implants. Most ENT programs are 5 years and include 1 or 2 years of preliminary surgery. A few of the more prestigious, heavily academic programs add another year for research. Many ENT graduates pursue fellowship training in one of a number of subspecialty fields, including head and neck surgery, laryngology, otology, neurotology, rhinology, and plastic and reconstructive surgery.

## Match Numbers

Otolaryngology continues to be an extremely competitive specialty. Both supply and demand have been steady: last year there were 386 applicants for 244 positions (Figure 3–11A). For the past two years all positions that were offered were filled (Figure 3–11B). In fact, the fill rate has remained near 100% for over 10 years (Figure 3–11B). The rate of U.S. seniors who did not match was down to 17% in 2000 from 25% in 1999 (Figure 3–11C). This continues the trend over the past several years of a declining unmatched rate for U.S. seniors. However, international medical graduates fared much worse, with a 94% non-match rate, up from 90% last year (Figure 3–11B).

## Application Tips

Strong applicants in this specialty have impressive all-around credentials, including research experience. USMLE Step 1 scores are often used by program directors as a screening tool, with some ENT applicants reporting cutoffs between the 75th and 85th percentiles. A recent study found a strong correlation between high medical school GPAs (if available), high board scores, high class rank (if available), honors in both junior surgery and medicine, and AΩA selection and ENT matching success. Some of the very competitive ENT programs suggest doing an audition rotation at their hospital to increase your likelihood of being invited for an interview. Otherwise, it's a good idea to do externships if you are aiming for specific programs where your application is less competitive than you'd like.

The average number of applications per student has risen dramatically over the past decade, from 12 in 1985 to an average of 33 in 1995. Unfortunately, the number of available positions and the number of interviews offered have largely remained unchanged.

Because there are only about 100 programs in ENT and only a few spots per program, you are operating at a serious disadvantage if you have to apply in a particular geographic region. Virtually all ENT applicants complete the 9-page universal ENT application, which must be received by a Central Application Service by mid-September. On the last page of this form, there is room to attach the names and addresses of the programs to which you want the application forwarded. The more programs you apply to, the higher the cost. Be sure to emphasize any research experience in your application. You are allowed to submit no more than three letters of recommendation. The most balanced approach is to submit two letters from ENT faculty and one from a clinical attending from another major clerkship (eg, medicine, OB/GYN, etc). The easiest advice to follow? **Never** use the collo-

Positions offered in otolaryngology and number filled.

Percentage of otolaryngology positions filled on Match Day.

**"ENT" IS A FOUR LETTER WORD TO MANY OTOLARYNGOLOGISTS.**

**FIGURE 3-11C**

OTOLARYNGOLOGY

Percentage of U.S. seniors unmatched in otolaryngology on Match Day.

quial term "ENT" in your application or interview visit; always say "otolaryngology."

## Interview Tips

Most ENT interviews are scheduled in November and December. If you're offered an interview at one program, it would not hurt to call other programs nearby where you have applied and ask if they are willing to grant you an interview while you are in the area. Most ENT programs, however, have only two to three interview dates per season. As a result, clustering interviews is often very difficult. Be ready to criss-cross the country to get all the interviews you need.

An applicant will typically sit for four to six interviews during the visit, each lasting 15 to 30 minutes. This schedule usually includes an interview with the department chairperson. Emphasize the strengths and interests you can offer that are most compatible with the philosophy of the particular program. It is always a good idea to highlight your academic and research interests when you are interviewed by the department chair, even if the program is more clinically oriented. Moreover, feel free to drop names, assuming that the interview is going well and that you are well liked by the people whose names you drop. ENT is a small field where anyone who's anyone knows everyone.

Note that if you are a competitive candidate, programs may try to ask you how you are ranking them. If that program is **not** your top choice, then tell the interviewer(s) that you regard their program highly but cannot in fairness make that decision until you have finished your interviews. If the program turns out to be one of your top choices, feel free to mention that fact in your follow-up thank-you letter.

## For More Info . . .

American Academy of Otolaryngology—
Head and Neck Surgery (AAO-HNS)
1 Prince Street
Alexandria, VA 22314
(703) 836-4444
http://www.entnch.org

American Academy of Facial Plastic and Reconstructive Surgery
(AAFPRS)
310 S. Henry Street
Alexandria, Virginia 22314
(703) 299-9291
(800) 332-FACE
http://www.facial-plastic-surgery.org

American Board of Otolaryngology
3050 Post Oak Boulevard, Suite 1700
Houston, Texas 77056
Voice: (713) 850-0399
Fax: (713) 850-1104
http://www.aboto.org

Association for Research in Otolaryngology
http://www.aro.org

San Francisco Match Otolaryngology Matching Program
PO Box 7584
San Francisco, CA 94120-7584
Phone: (415) 447-0350
Fax: (415) 561-8535
E-mail: help@sfmatch.org
http://www.sfmatch.org

National Meetings

AAO-HNS Foundation 2000 Annual Meeting
September 24 through 27, 2000 in Washington, DC

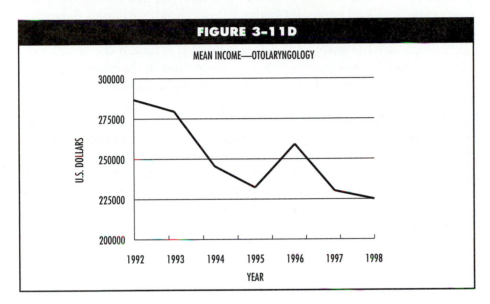

Mean income of otolaryngologists in U.S. dollars.

# PATHOLOGY

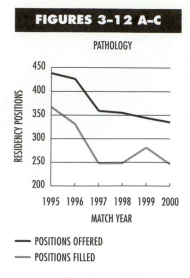

PATHOLOGY

— POSITIONS OFFERED
— POSITIONS FILLED

Positions offered in pathology and number filled.

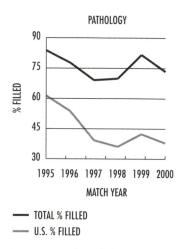

PATHOLOGY

— TOTAL % FILLED
— U.S. % FILLED

Percentage of pathology positions filled on Match Day.

PATHOLOGY

Percentage of U.S. seniors unmatched in pathology on Match Day.

Because of the rise in surgical and needle biopsies as part of the diagnostic process, pathologists are becoming more active in direct patient care. The downside of the specialty, however, continues to be an increase in the number of government and laboratory regulations, which result in more paperwork, less time for actual patient care, decreased funding for research programs, and curtailed patient contact compared with other fields. Specialists currently in the work force find that they have to work longer hours for the same pay. Furthermore, private practices are not hiring as many pathologists, especially in large urban centers. As a result, more residents are delaying graduation from the training programs and choosing instead to take 1 or 2 extra years to acquire more distinctive fellowship skills to make themselves desirable to potential employers. Many are also choosing research as an alternative to hospital practice. It is still unclear at this time if the trend of decreasing job opportunities in pathology will continue in the future.

To be board-qualified in either anatomic or clinical pathology requires a minimum of 4 years. Entering students should look at combined programs, which offer a 5-year residency covering both types of pathology giving you a sort of "bilingual" appeal. Certified in one specialty, you might be limited to working in large hospitals that can afford to employ separate specialists.

Pathology training is relatively flexible, as long as the resident completes the core rotations required for board certifications, such as surgical pathology, cytopathology, autopsy, and subspecialty rotations particular to each emphasis. He or she is then free to take elective courses, conduct research, or acquire further training in a specialized area of interest, such as forensic pathology.

## Match Numbers

In spite of improved recognition, the field of pathology still suffers from a shortage of qualified applicants. Over the past five years, the number of positions offered by pathology programs have decreased slightly each year (Figure 3–12A). In the same time period, the number of positions filled have also decreased. In 2000, only 246 of the 335 positions offered, or 73.4% were filled through the NRMP Match (Figures 3–12A and 3–12B). With the large number of unfilled positions in pathology, students usually are able to match into the pathology program of their choice. Given the possible decline in job prospects, pathology programs will continue to cut the number of positions offered.

## Application Tips

Because training programs in pathology have different emphases, it is important to find one that matches your career goals. This is especially true for combined clinical and anatomic pathology programs, which may be strong in only one department. After you select your emphasis, the next step is to demonstrate your desire to enter the field of pathology to the programs of your choice. A strong evaluation in the senior elective, accompanied by solid letters of recommendation (at least one from a pathologist), is essential in this process. Most programs use their own application forms instead of the Universal Application supplied by the NRMP, so be sure to request the appropriate information and forms early. Application material should be completed as soon as possible, preferably by mid-November.

## Interview Tips

Given the less than glamorous image of pathology, most interviewers will be extremely curious to know why you are interested in the field. Be prepared to answer many questions about your particular interests, any research background, or any plans for your future career. Interviews often last about 30 minutes, with three to six interviews a day, depending on whether you are applying to the combined or single program. In general, pathology interviews are relaxed, with only occasional tough questions. Expect to answer some questions about your post-residency plans, such as research, extra training, or going straight into private practice.

If you are ranked highly by a pathology program, you can expect some pressure to rank the program highly in return. Contrary to the official Match guidelines, many program directors will contact strong applicants and question them about their rankings. Be sure to keep your cool and not be pressured into making a "commitment" prematurely.

## For More Info . . .

▶ *Student Information Packet.* This free packet includes several articles and a slick brochure about career opportunities in pathology. The College of American Pathologists also produces a promotional video that it lends out at no cost. To receive an information packet or borrow the video, call or write:

> College of American Pathologists (CAP)
> 325 Waukegan Road
> North Field, IL 60093
> (800) 323-4040
> http://www.cap.org

▶ American Society of Clinical Pathologists (ASCP)
> 2100 West Harrison Street
> Chicago, IL 60612-3798
> (312) 738-1336
> http://www.ascp.org

National Meetings
> ASCP/CAP 2000 Annual Meeting and Exhibits
> October 14 through 19, 2000 at the San Diego Marriott Hotel
>   in San Diego, CA

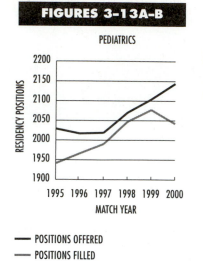

**FIGURES 3-13A-B**

PEDIATRICS

POSITIONS OFFERED
POSITIONS FILLED

Positions offered in pediatrics and number filled.

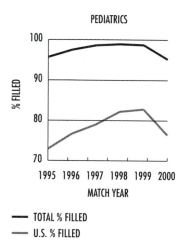

PEDIATRICS

TOTAL % FILLED
U.S. % FILLED

Percentage of pediatrics positions filled on Match Day.

**MOST APPLICANTS WHO DID NOT GET INTERVIEWS SIMPLY APPLIED TOO LATE.**

## PEDIATRICS

Pediatrics has a reputation as an easygoing specialty. Satisfied pediatricians enjoy developing relationships with their young patients as they grow up. Unlike family physicians, pediatricians can evaluate the whole family without being responsible for every member's medical care. Today the field is seeing more routine procedures and well-child care done by nurse practitioners, physician assistants, and family practitioners, which means pediatricians can focus on the care of the seriously ill. The trend in residency training favors increased ambulatory care. The current health care climate assures excellent employment prospects for pediatricians. In addition, preventive health care, an integral part of pediatrics, will be encouraged. However, the long arm of managed care is threatening to squeeze pediatric subspecialists and the population of children's hospitals, which have high operating expenses because of the nature of their training mission.

Pediatric programs can be roughly classified by setting: children's versus non-children's hospital. Children's hospitals have more pediatrics specialists available and in general offer more comprehensive training and education. In a children's hospital, everything is geared toward kids, from the intubating equipment in the ER to the wallpaper in the CT units. Children's hospitals tend to be located in large cities and have more of a tertiary care focus. Good children's hospitals have affiliations with adult centers for delivery room experience.

By contrast, residencies in non-children's hospitals provide more interaction with faculty and house staff from other primary care specialties that involve children, such as family practice, OB/GYN and internal medicine. These programs can be further categorized into community, university, and county/municipal settings. These are discussed in more detail in Chapter 4.

### Match Numbers

The number of positions filled in pediatrics decreased in 2000 for the first time in the past 10 years (Figure 3-13A). In the 2000 Match, 95.2% of the 2144 available pediatric positions were filled, down from 98.7% in 1999 (Figures 3-13A and 3-13B). At the same time, the number of positions filled by international medical graduates increased from 15.9% in 1999 to 18.8% in 2000 (Figure 3-13B). The interest in pediatrics seems to be declining as there has been a decrease in the fill rate and a concurrent decrease in the total unmatched rate from 3.7% in 1999 to 2.7% in 2000 (Figure 3-13C).

### Application Tips

Though pediatrics is on the upswing, securing an interview is still mostly a matter of scheduling, since most programs do not seriously screen applicants. In fact, many programs ask the applicant to call in automatically after submitting the application to schedule an interview. Therefore, we strongly advise that you submit your applications when programs first accept them in the early fall. Do not be one of the many qualified applicants who get locked out of interviews each year because of poor timing. Though the number of applications you should submit depends on your strength as a candidate and the programs to which you are applying, most applicants are generally advised to submit 10 to 15 applications.

It goes without saying that your personal statement and CV should emphasize any involvement with children, community or public health care, or volunteer activity. As in the other primary care specialties, the type of individual you are and your long-term goals will provide fodder for question-and-answer sessions.

## Interview Tips

Most interviews for pediatrics programs are scheduled from late November through January. The interview day typically runs from 8 AM to 3 PM. Expect two to four interview sessions, 20 to 45 minutes in length. Interviews in this specialty are generally low-key and non-confrontational. In addition to having the qualities typically desired in all house officers, you must package yourself as an individual who interacts well with parents and children. Good interpersonal skills are a must. Remember that most of your interviewers are parents themselves.

## For More Info . . .

► *Pediatrics Information Packet.* In addition to a general profile of the specialty, this packet includes fact sheets detailing current socioeconomic statistics on pediatric practice. To receive this information, gratis, call or write:

> American Academy of Pediatrics (AAP)
> 141 Northwest Point Blvd
> Elk Grove Village, IL 60007
> (800) 433-9016, ext. 7914 or
> (708) 228-5005, ext. 7914
> http://www.aap.org

► *Selecting a Pediatric Residency: An Employment Guide.* This is a comprehensive, step-by-step guide to selecting, applying to, and interviewing at pediatric residency programs. It also discusses family and marriage considerations, such employment issues as contract and salary guidelines, and certification licensing requirements. It's available to medical students for $5 plus shipping costs. To order, call or write:

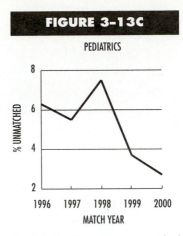

### FIGURE 3-13C

PEDIATRICS

Percentage of U.S. seniors unmatched in pediatrics on Match Day.

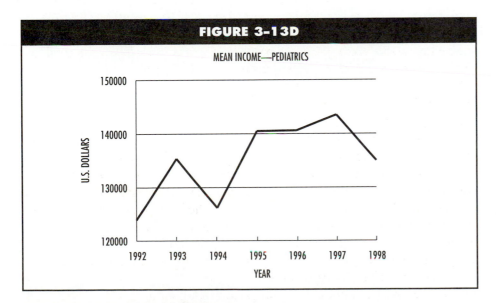

### FIGURE 3-13D

MEAN INCOME—PEDIATRICS

Mean income of pediatrician in U.S. dollars.

AAP, Publications Department
PO Box 927
Elk Grove Village, IL 60009-0927
(800) 433-9016

► Kappy, M: The pediatric residency program of the future: I. The changing face of today's private pediatric practice. *Am J Dis Child* 1987; 141:945. Though somewhat dated, this series of articles addresses many issues that remain current in pediatrics.

► Kappy, M: The pediatric residency program of the future: II. Tomorrow's private pediatric practice: A change in roles. *Am J Dis Child* 1987; 141:1045.

► Kappy, M: The pediatric residency program of the future: III. Modifying pediatric residency training programs. *Am J Dis Child* 1987;141:1156.

National Meetings

Advancing Children's Health 2000: A Joint Meeting of the Pediatric Academic Societies (PAS) and the American Academy of Pediatrics (AAP)

May 12 through 16, 2000 in Boston, Massachusetts (visit www.aps-spr.org for more information)

American Academy of Pediatrics Annual Meeting

October 28 through November 1, 2000 in Chicago, Illinois

# PHYSICAL MEDICINE AND REHABILITATION

Physical medicine and rehabilitation (PM&R), also known as physiatry, is concerned with the diagnosis, evaluation and treatment of patients with limited function secondary to disease, injury, impairment and/or disabilities. PM&R physicians take a holistic approach to patient diagnosis and treatment, thereby focusing on physical, social, psychological and vocational function. PM&R physicians also concentrate on health maintenance, prevention of secondary complications and alleviation of pain. Physiatrists are trained in therapeutic exercise, physical modalities, prosthetics, orthotics, gait analysis, diagnostic and therapeutic injections, electrodiagnostic studies; and rehabilitation management. They practice in rehabilitation centers, hospitals and private offices. Physical medicine and rehabilitation physicians are able to make and maintain relationships with their patients, see a wide variety of patient problems and enjoy a comfortable lifestyle often with little or no night call. However, PM&R physicians are frustrated by difficulties encountered in patient treatment.

Residency training is one year in a transitional program, followed by three years in a physical medicine & rehabilitation training program. Residents may choose to spend their first year divided into six months in a transitional year program and six months in a family practice, internal medicine, pediatrics, or surgery or any combination of these patient care experiences.

## Match Numbers

Physical medicine and rehabilitation has not been a very competitive specialty in recent years, with a total fill rate ranging from 70 to 85% in recent years (Figure 3–14B). However there are only a small number of programs, and there has been a decline in the number of positions offered each year (Figure 3–14A). The decrease in available spots has made this specialty slightly more competitive than it once was. Nevertheless, the unmatch rate in 2000 was 0%, significantly lower than the 4.6% unmatch rate in 1999 (Figure 3–14C). The number of positions filled by international medical graduates is growing each year, with an all time high of 45.4% in 1999 (Figure 3–14B).

## Application Tips

Physical medicine and rehabilitation is relatively less competitive than other fields, making it more of a buyers market. Applicants should consider different programs to evaluate which programs are most compatible with their career goals. Personal statements should demonstrate a clear reason for your interest in the specialty and if possible demonstrate past experiences. Applications should be submitted by mid-October. You should apply to 10 to 15 programs and interview at 8 to 10.

## Interview Tips

Interviews tend to be personal and humanistic, often with the interviewer curious as to how the applicant became interested in physical medicine and rehabilitation. Expect approximately two to four interviews.

**FIGURES 3–14A–C**

Positions offered in physical medicine and rehabilitation (PM&R) and number filled.

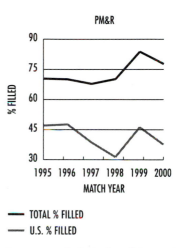

Percentage of physical medicine and rehabilitation (PM&R) positions filled on Match Day.

Percentage of U.S. seniors unmatched in physical medicine and rehabilitation (PM&R) on Match Day.

American Academy of Physical Medicine and Rehabilitation
   (AAPM&R)
One IBM Plaza, Suite 2500
Chicago, IL 60611-3604
Phone: (312) 464-9700
Fax: (312) 464-0227
http://www.aapmr.org

National Meetings

AAPM&R 62nd Annual Assembly and Technical Exhibition
November 2 through 5, 2000 at the Hilton San Francisco and Towers
   in San Francisco, CA

# PSYCHIATRY

The widespread shift toward primary care has affected psychiatry in several ways. Issues often mentioned include lack of adequate provision for mental health care by most insurance plans or HMOs. The shift of psychotherapeutic care to primary care physicians, psychologists, and social workers also cuts into the available work for board-certified psychiatrists. Although practitioners report a high satisfaction rate with the work involved—and the mean income in this field has been relatively steady (Figure 3–15D)—many also register anxiety about the future of the specialty.

Residencies in psychiatry generally require 1 year of internship, preferably in preliminary medicine, followed by 3 years of training in psychiatry. Some have a fourth year with emphasis in neurology or geriatrics. Depending on the program, training can emphasize either psychotherapy or the biological aspects of mental illness. Thus, it is important to determine whether the orientation of a particular program matches your expectations and field of interest.

## Match Numbers

Applications in psychiatry have increased over the past five to six years, making the specialty somewhat more difficult to enter relative to the easy nature of matching several years ago. In 2000, 893 of the 996 available positions, or 89.7% were filled through the NRMP Match (Figures 3–15A and 3–15B). The rate of unmatched students is low compared to other specialties, with 3.1% and 3.3% of applicants unmatched in 2000 and 1999 respectively (Figure 3–15C).

## Application Tips

Unlike other fields, personal statements for psychiatry are traditionally substantial in length (two-page personal statements are OK) and should discuss in some detail your interest in and understanding of the field. Except for a few prestigious programs, most do not pay much attention to board scores. Rather, emphasis is placed on the applicant's clinical evaluations, especially in psychiatry rotations. Good letters of recommendation, as well as documented interests in the field, such as prior research or involvement in mental health care, will further strengthen your application. Again, early completion of application material is important. The average number of applications submitted ranges from 10 to 15, with about 8 to 10 interviews recommended.

## Interview Tips

During the interview day, the applicant has an average of 4 interviews, lasting 45 to 60 minutes each. Questions tend to probe the applicant's desire to enter psychiatry and his or her ability to interact with other people. It's a good idea to review strengths and weaknesses ahead of time, since many of the questions may deal with your personality. Some applicants compare these interviews to psychoanalytical sessions placing you on the proverbial couch. Little or no pimping is involved, except regarding the candidate's previous research experience. In general, expect to meet psychiatrists who seek potential colleagues with stable personalities and good interpersonal

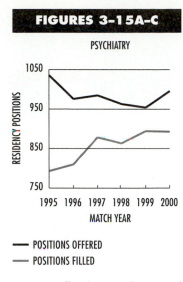

POSITIONS OFFERED
POSITIONS FILLED

Positions offered in psychiatry and number filled.

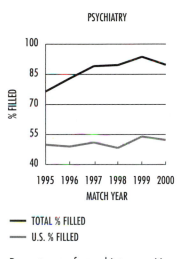

TOTAL % FILLED
U.S. % FILLED

Percentage of psychiatry positions filled on Match Day.

Percentage of U.S. seniors unmatched in psychiatry on Match Day.

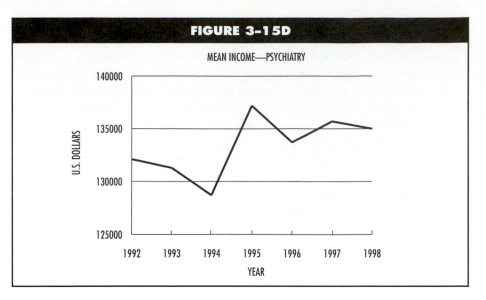

**FIGURE 3-15D**

MEAN INCOME—PSYCHIATRY

Mean income of psychiatrists in U.S. dollars.

skills. According to experienced applicants, an unspoken purpose of the interview is to rule out obvious psychopathology.

**ONE PURPOSE OF THE INTERVIEW IS TO RULE OUT OBVIOUS PSYCHOPATHOLOGY.**

## For More Info . . .

▶ *Directory of Psychiatric Residency Training Programs.* Although this directory is not updated as often as AMA-FREIDA, it has a more logical, user-friendly format. Information unique to the directory includes contact name and number for student electives, house staff contact names, and diagrams of a typical resident rotation schedule. The directory also offers general advice about residency applications. It's available at your psychiatry department or can be ordered for $25 with a student discount from:

American Psychiatric Press, Inc.
1400 K Street NW
Washington, DC 20005
(800) 368-5777

American Psychiatric Association (APA)
1400 K. Street NW
Washington, DC 20005
Phone: (202) 682-6000
http://www.psych.org

American Academy of Child Psychiatry (AACAP)
3615 Wisconsin Avenue NW
Washington, DC 20016
Phone: (202) 966-7300
http://www.aacap.org

National Meetings

American Psychiatric Association Annual Meeting
May 13 through 18, 2000 in Chicago, IL

## RADIOLOGY

Radiology is a field that has grown tremendously in the last decade, thanks primarily to technological advances in imaging techniques. Radiologists continue to enjoy a good lifestyle, relatively high income (Figure 3–16D), and flexible work hours. The advent of managed care, however, and the focus on primary care pose worrisome trends for the field. Practitioners in other fields, such as cardiology, gastroenterology, and urology, are performing many imaging guided procedures. Employment, especially in large cities with a high density of MDs, is increasingly difficult to find. Many hospitals are hiring fewer radiologists, thus making the ones already employed work longer hours. Cutbacks in trained technologists and ancillary personnel in the radiology department also cause increased workloads and heavier paperwork.

Training in radiology generally requires 1 year of internship followed by 4 years of diagnostic radiology. The internship year can be satisfied by completion of a transitional, surgical, or preliminary medicine year. The style of radiology training depends on the institution, but all institutions will cover the major imaging modalities, including nuclear medicine. Post-residency fellowships (1 to 2 years) are offered in a wide variety of organ-based specialties, including neuroimaging, vascular/interventional, mammography/women's imaging, body imaging, chest, and musculoskeletal; and in modality-based fellowships, such as computed tomography, magnetic resonance, ultrasonography, and nuclear medicine.

### Match Numbers

The application to radiology residency programs is more competitive now than ever before. The number of positions offered by radiology programs was dramatically reduced from 1996 to 1997 by 23% from 1154 to 890 (Figure 3–16A). The radiology residency positions offered have continued to decline since then, with a total of 841 spots offered in 2000 (Figure 3–16A). As expected, the fill rates have risen over this time period, with 98.7% of positions being filled in 2000, up from 60.9% in 1996 (Figure 3–16B). The unmatched rates have also risen extensively over the past several years, up from 8.2% in 1999 to 14.1% in 2000, a much higher rate than the 1.4% unmatched rate seen in 1997 (Figure 3–16C).

### Application Tips

Strong evaluations in the senior clinical rotations, especially radiology, support the successful application. High board scores and excellent letters of recommendation by senior radiology faculty members are next in importance. Research experience or a technical background prior to entering medical school is viewed favorably. As with other competitive specialties, early completion of application material is important. You will need to be well-organized to coordinate applications for both internship and residency positions. Although the competitiveness of the applicants may be declining, applicants are usually advised to submit 15 to 20 in order to obtain a comfortable 10 to 15 interviews.

### Interview Tips

Because of the small number of spots available, residency programs in radiology tend to offer interviews only to strong applicants in whom they are seriously interested. Each candidate's visit typically includes two to five interviews, 15 to 30 minutes in length. Interviews for radiology often tend to be

UNDERSTAND THE DIFFERENCES BETWEEN DIAGNOSTIC RADIOLOGY, NUCLEAR MEDICINE, AND RADIATION ONCOLOGY.

## FIGURES 3-16 A-B

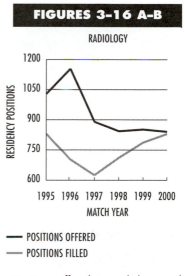

Positions offered in radiology and number filled.

Percentage of radiology positions filled on Match Day.

**FIGURE 3-16C**

Percentage of U.S. seniors unmatched in radiology on Match Day.

**TABLE 3–2. Most commonly asked interview questions in Radiology.**

| Interview Question | % of Applicants Who Received Question |
|---|---|
| Why are you going into radiology? | 71% |
| Why did you apply here or why do you want to come here? | 32% |
| What do you see yourself doing in the future? | 23% |
| Are you applying to other programs? If so, what are they? | 23% |
| Why should we choose you? | 16% |
| What do you do in your spare time? | 13% |
| Name your strengths and weaknesses. | 13% |
| Do you have any questions? | 13% |
| How did you become interested in radiology? | 10% |

relaxed, placing the major emphasis on the applicant's reason for entering the field and interviewing at this particular institution (Table 3–2). You might be invited to attend a clinical case conference, but almost no one expects you to be able to read an x-ray on the spot. Quantifying a "good eye" in radiology is even harder than evaluating manual dexterity for a surgical field, so programs don't even try.

The interviewers will also attempt to predict how well you can relate to other professionals, since much of radiology consists of consulting work (ie, being a "doctor's doctor"). In general, these sessions are low-stress, with little or no pimping involved. Let the program showcase its strengths; don't ask questions that highlight its weaknesses. For example, if they don't have a $5 million high-field research magnet, don't ask about the (im)possibility of their buying one for you. On the other hand, if they have one, feel free to discuss its relevance to your research.

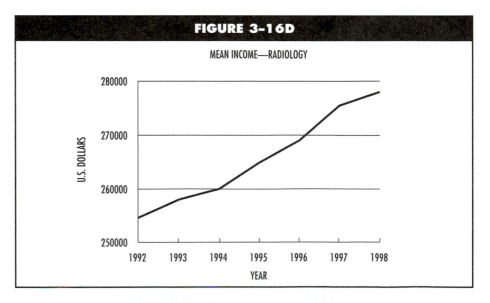

Mean income of radiology in U.S. dollars.

## For More Info . . .

▶ *Career Information Packet.* This packet includes a brochure describing the field of radiology as well as several articles describing the job prospects, average earnings, and practice characteristics. This information can be obtained free of charge by calling or writing:

> American College of Radiology (ACR)
> 1891 Preston White Drive
> Reston, VA 22091
> (800) ACR-LINE
> (703) 648-8900
> http://www.acr.org

National Meetings

> American College of Radiology (ACR) Annual Meeting
> September 23 through 27, 2000 at the New York Hilton
>     and Towers, New York, NY
> For more information, contact:
> Mary Jane Donahue at (703) 648-8902

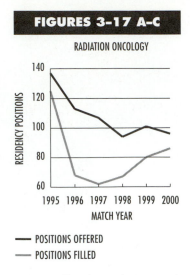

RADIATION ONCOLOGY

Positions offered in radiation oncology and number filled.

RADIATION ONCOLOGY

Percentage of radiation oncology positions filled on Match Day.

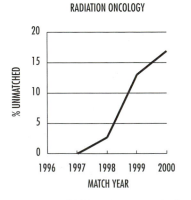

RADIATION ONCOLOGY

Percentage of U.S. seniors unmatched in radiation oncology on Match Day.

# RADIATION ONCOLOGY

Radiation oncologists are an essential part of the multidisciplinary management of cancer patients, collaborating closely with other physicians in the management of cancer patients. Radiation oncology uses radiation therapy in the treatment of patients with cancer and other diseases. Radiation oncology is an attractive field to many because of the relatively easy lifestyle with minimal call duties. As a result this field is becoming more and more competitive.

A one year internship in either internal medicine or transitional year is required for this specialty, followed by four years of residency in radiation oncology.

## Match Results

This field has recently become much more competitive than it once was. There are few programs that offer training positions in radiation oncology, and with the increased interest in this specialty, there has been a surge in the number of unmatched students (Figure 3–17C). Although there were no unmatched students as recently as 1997, 16.9% of applicants were unmatched in 2000, up from 13% unmatched in 1999 (Figure 3–17C). The majority of positions are filled by U.S. seniors.

## Application Tips

With the increasing competitiveness of radiation oncology, applicants should do their best to have a strong application to increase their chances of matching. Factors that increase the opportunity to match in competitive programs include AΩA status and high USMLE scores. Strong letters of recommendation from internal medicine and radiation oncology are essential. Applicants should submit 10 to 15 applications to undergo 8 to 10 interviews.

## Interview Tips

Interviews are usually conducted on an individual basis. Expect three to four interviews, lasting approximately 30 minutes each. Issues that may be touched upon during the interview are death, dying and euthanasia in order for the program to assess your ability to address end of life issues.

## For More Info . . .

American College of Radiation Oncology (ACRO)
820 Jorie Boulevard
Oak Brook, IL 60523
Phone: (630) 368-3733
Fax: (630) 571-7837
http://www.acro.org

American Society for Therapeutic Radiology and Oncology (ASTRO)
12500 Fair Lakes Circle
Suite 375
Fairfax, VA 22033-3882
Phone: (800) 962-7876, (703) 502-1550
Fax: (703) 502-7852
http://www.astro.org

National Meetings

The 10th Annual Meeting of the American College of Radiation Oncology
May 6 through 7, 2000 at The Park Hyatt in Washington, DC

# SURGERY

General surgery residencies have increased in popularity over the past few years, thus making the field increasingly competitive for aspiring surgeons. The specialty boasts a number of benefits: the chance to apply technical and procedural skills toward quick resolutions of medical problems, good doctor/patient relationships, and relatively high income (Figure 3–18D). Drawbacks include long hours, rigorous training, increasing paperwork, and the intrusion of such prickly non-clinical issues as malpractice liability, government regulations, and third-party payers. Generally, most surgeons remain highly satisfied with their work, notwithstanding the changes they make in their practices to accommodate HMOs and other complications.

Surgical residencies require a minimum of 5 years of training, with some programs requiring as many as 3 additional research years. These often come in the middle or later portion of the residency, at a time when residents can also moonlight. Subspecialty training includes critical care surgery, hand surgery, pediatric surgery, plastic surgery, vascular surgery, and trauma surgery.

## Match Numbers

Surgery remains very competitive. In 2000, 1008 of the 1023 positions available were filled through the NRMP on Match Day, resulting in a 98.5% fill rate (Figures 3–18A, 3–18B). The number of positions offered and number filled has remained stable, however the unmatched rate of students has dropped from 18.7 in 1996 to 7.3% in 2000 (Figure 3–18C). In general, the majority, on average approximately 86%, of applicants matching in general surgery programs are U.S. senior medical students.

## Application Tips

Before applying, you should think about whether you would be happier in a clinical or a research-oriented program, noting that length of training varies from one type of program to the other. Generally, strong evaluations in the senior surgical rotations are essential to successful applications. The *pièce de résistance* would be a strong letter from the chief of surgery. Programs with an academic slant will definitely consider the applicant's research background fundamental to the evaluation process, whereas those with a clinical focus will attempt to determine the applicant's potential to be a good surgeon. For advice and connection purposes, it's always helpful to find a mentor who is well known in the field. As with other competitive residencies, early completion of application material is important. Although the desired number of applications depends on the applicant's quality, the average ranges from 15 to 20, with a goal of at least 10 to 12 interviews suggested.

## Interview Tips

As one applicant put it, the interview is used mainly to eliminate malignant personalities. They may be tolerated at the attending level, but no one wants to deal with this problem in a junior resident. Interview committees often have a good idea of how they are going to rank you before they even meet you. Interview days are usually Saturdays and often consist of 2 to 3 sessions, lasting 30 to 45 minutes each. Occasionally, one is asked to present a clinical case or to discuss how to deal with the stress of a surgical residency. Often, interviews are laid-back, with little or no pimping. However, academic programs tend to opt for more pointed questions, inquiring about your research

GENERAL SURGERY

— POSITIONS OFFERED
— POSITIONS FILLED

Positions offered in surgery and number filled.

GENERAL SURGERY

— TOTAL % FILLED
— U.S. % FILLED

Percentage of general surgery positions filled on Match Day.

GENERAL SURGERY

Percentage of U.S. seniors unmatched in general surgery on Match Day.

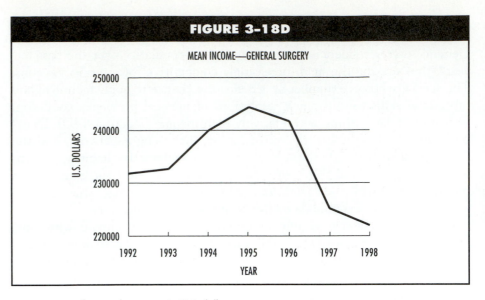

**FIGURE 3-18D**

MEAN INCOME—GENERAL SURGERY

Mean income of general surgeons in U.S. dollars.

background and any current projects. Try to learn something about the program's reputation for research.

## For More Info . . .

▶ Johansen K, Heimbach DM: *So You Want to Be a Surgeon . . . A Medical Student Guide to Finding and Matching With the Best Possible Residency*. This book includes a brief but very helpful discussion of surgical residency applications. The greater part of the book is devoted to descriptions of most of the surgery programs in the United States and Puerto Rico. The authors attempt to classify programs by the caliber of the house staff. The book is in some medical bookstores, and can also be ordered for about $12 from:

> Educational Clearinghouse
> Department of Surgery
> Southern Illinois University
>    School of Medicine
> PO Box 19230
> Springfield, IL 62794
> (217) 785-3835

▶ *The Surgical Career Handbook*. This glossy booklet provides an overview of surgery and profiles its subspecialties. The information, however, is often too general to be useful. This publication is available for $7 from:

> American College of Surgeons
> 633 N. St. Clair Street
> Chicago, IL 60611
> (312) 202-5000
> http://www.facs.org

More information can be obtained from:

American College of Chest Physicians
3300 Dundee Road
Northbrook, IL 60062
(847) 498-1400
http://www.chestnet.org

American College of Colon and Rectal Surgeons
85 West Algonquin Road, Suite 550
Arlington Heights, IL 60005
Phone: (847) 290-9184
http://www.fascrs.org

National Meetings

American College of Surgeons Spring Meeting
April 30 through May 3, 2000 in Washington, DC
2000 Clinical Congress
October 22 through 27, 2000 in Chicago, IL

TRANSITIONAL YEAR

— POSITIONS OFFERED
— POSITIONS FILLED

Positions offered in transitional year programs (TYP) and number filled.

TRANSITIONAL YEAR

— TOTAL % FILLED
— U.S. % FILLED

Percentage of transitional year program (TYP) positions filled on Match Day.

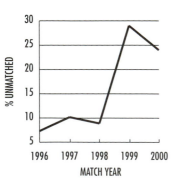

TRANSITIONAL YEAR

Percentage of U.S. seniors unmatched in transitional year programs (TYP) on Match Day.

# TRANSITIONAL YEAR PROGRAM (TYP)

For those on a quest for a flexible internship, TYPs continue to be a popular choice. In contrast to the preliminary medicine or preliminary surgery years, transitional internships allow for exposure to many other fields, such as OB/GYN, ER, orthopedics, pediatrics, anesthesia, as well as traditional medicine and surgery. Transitional internships consist of multiple rotations through different departments. The length of each rotation, and the type of work involved are usually extremely flexible and can be tailored to fit each individual's need. Some programs, however, will have certain required core rotations that must be satisfied. In general, the requirements are minimal and can be easily fulfilled. The variety of experience is ideal for anyone entering a residency, such as emergency medicine, in which a wide base of knowledge is desirable.

Other students take a TYP because they're undecided on a specialty, but this can prove a difficult undertaking. By the time your year starts, the application process is already upon you. In addition, finding time for interviews during the year can be impossible. Make sure you reach an understanding with the program director/chief resident regarding time you will need to apply and interview. If you can't take sufficient time off, you may be better off taking a year off for research or an MPH.

## Match Numbers

Although TYPs were not considered competitive in the past, the number of unmatched students has risen dramatically over the past several years (Figure 3–19C). The number of positions offered by programs has declined over time from 1337 in 1994 to 1005 in 2000 (Figure 3–19A). In 2000, 944 of 1005 positions, or 94% of available positions were filled (Figure 3–19B). Also, the number of positions filled by international medical graduates have decreased substantially from 25% in 1996 to approximately 12% in 2000 (Figure 3–19B). The unmatched rate of U.S. senior medical students was 24% in 2000, slightly lower than the 29% of students unmatched in 1999, but still dramatically increased from the relatively low 7.3% unmatched in 1996 (Figure 3–19C).

## Application Tips

As with most internship programs, the competitiveness of the program depends on the reputation of the institution and the flexibility of the program. Applicants should have strong clinical evaluations, strong letters of recommendation, and convincing reasons for seeking a transitional internship. Board scores tend to be less important, except at very prestigious institutions. Early submission of application material is important. The recommended deadline is early November, despite the February date posted by many programs.

## Interview Tips

Interviews are casually conducted and are even optional for some programs. Usually, the applicant will be scheduled for 2 or 3 sessions, lasting 30 minutes each. Questions try to appraise the candidate's ability to fit in with the program, his or her desire for a transitional residency, and post-internship plans. Some transitional medicine residency directors do not like having their program used as "down time" for consideration of career plans, so be prepared to discuss your long-term career goals.

# For More Info . . .

▶ *Transitional Year Program Directory*. More popularly known as the "Purple Book." This annually updated directory is available at your student affairs office. You can order your own copy by calling or writing:

Association for Hospital Medical Education
Council of Transitional Year Program Directors
1200 19th Street NW, Suite 300
Washington, DC 20035-2401
(202) 857-1196

▶ Kimball Mohn, MD
Chair of the Council of Transitional Year Program Directors
Mercy Hospital, Department of Medicine
1400 Locust Street
Pittsburgh, PA 15219
(412) 232-8080

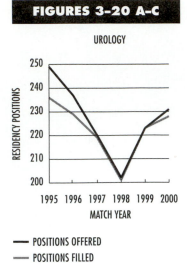

UROLOGY

■ POSITIONS OFFERED
■ POSITIONS FILLED

Positions offered in urology and number filled.

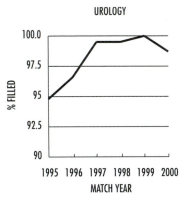

UROLOGY

■ TOTAL % FILLED

Percentage of urology positions filled on Match Day.

UROLOGY

Percentage of U.S. seniors unmatched in urology on Match Day.

# UROLOGY

Urology is the medical and surgical specialty that deals with disorders of the male and female urinary tract and the male reproductive organs. Urologists see patients with kidney, ureter, bladder, prostate, urethra and male genital structure disorders and injuries. They also investigate and treat infertility and male sexual dysfunction. Although generally classified as a surgical specialty, urology also encompasses knowledge of internal medicine, pediatrics, gynecology, and other specialties. Diagnostic procedures are routinely performed in this specialty, including endoscopic, percutaneous and open surgery to treat congenital and acquired disorders of the reproductive and urinary systems and related structures. Urologists enjoy seeing a variety of patients, and the combination of medicine and surgery in one specialty. As a result, urology is a popular and competitive field despite the rigors of its residency training.

Residency training involves one to two years of training in a general surgery program, followed by at least three to four years in a urology training program.

## Match Results

Urology is an extremely competitive specialty. The number of positions offered by programs has remained stable as has the number of applicants. In 2000, 228, or 98.7% of the 231 positions offered were filled (Figures 3–20A and 3–20B). In previous years, the total fill rate has been similarly high, often above 99% (Figure 3–20B). As expected, there is a high rate of unmatched applicants each year, with 24% of U.S. seniors unmatched in 2000, down from the 29% who were unmatched in 1999 (Figure 3–20C).

## Application Tips

Urology applications go through an early match. It is recommended that students submit their applications as soon as possible. Although the deadlines are November and December, applications should be mailed by October. Application factors which will make your application stronger include AΩA status, high USMLE 1 scores (above 80th percentile), high GPA (if applicable), strong evaluations, and a recommendation from the chief of urology. Research in urology certainly will make your application favor more positively.

## Interview Tips

Interviews may be conducted on a group or individual basis and are usually on a friendly and relaxed level. There are usually two to three interviews lasting 30 to 45 minutes each, attempting to ascertain your personality and whether or not it is compatible with theirs. Expect direct questions about your interest in clinical and/or research aspects of the program you are applying for.

## For More Info . . .

Listing of Accredited Urology Programs
Administrative Assistant, RRC for Urology
ACGME
515 N. State Street, Suite 2000
Chicago, IL 60610
(312) 464-5585

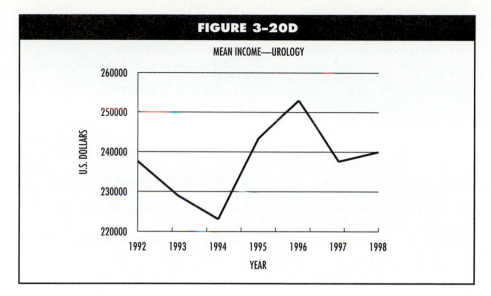

**FIGURE 3-20D**

MEAN INCOME—UROLOGY

Mean income of urologists in U.S. dollars.

American Board of Urology
2216 Ivy Road, Suite 210
Charlottesville, VA 22903
(804) 979-0059

American Urological Association Headquarters
1120 North Charles Street
Baltimore, MD 21201
Phone: (410) 727-1100
Fax: (410) 223-4370

American Urological Association (AUA) Office of Education
2425 West Loop South, Suite 333
Houston, TX 77027-4207
Phone: (800) 282-7077, (713) 622-2700
Fax: (713) 622-2898
http://www.auanet.org

AUA Residency Matching Program
2425 West Loop South
Suite 333
Houston, TX 77027-4207
Phone: (713) 622-2700, ext. 86
Fax: (713) 622-2898, (800) 282-7077, ext. 86
Vacancy Hotline: (800) 282-7077, ext. 88
http://www.auanet.org

National Meetings:

American Urological Association 95th Annual Meeting
April 29 through May 4, 2000 in Atlanta, GA

# REFERENCES

Baker JD et al: Selection of anesthesiology residents. *Acad Med* 1994;68:161.

Calhoun K et al: The resident selection process in otolaryngology—head and neck surgery. *Arch Otolaryngol Head Neck Surg* 1990;116:1041.

Center for Health Policy Research, *Physician Marketplace Statistics* 1994. Chicago: American Medical Association, 1994.

Center for Health Policy Research, *Physician Marketplace Statistics* 1994. Chicago: American Medical Association, 1998.

Center for Health Policy Research, *Socioeconomic Characteristics of Medical Practice 1995.* Chicago: American Medical Association, 1995.

Center for Health Policy Research, *Socioeconomic Characteristics of Medical Practice 1995.* Chicago: American Medical Association, 1999.

Ende J: The 1995 match: Internal medicine and other generalist specialties attract more US grads. *APDIM Newsletter*, March 1995.

Featherstone H, Ramsey P: Analysis of selection criteria for medical residents. *Am J Med* 1983;75.

Kahn NB, Graham R, Schmittling G: Entry of US medical school graduates into family practice residencies: 1991-1992 and 11-year summary. *Fam Med* 1992;24:504.

Kurtzke J et al: On the production of neurologists in the United States. *Neurology* 1991;41:1.

Medschool.com website (http://www.medschool.com).

NRMP, *Advanced Copy of Results and Data, 2000 Match.* Washington, DC, 2000.

NRMP, *1999 NRMP Data: April 1999.* Washington, DC, 1999.

NRMP, *1998 NRMP Data: 1998.* Washington, DC, 1998.

NRMP, *1997 NRMP Data: 1997.* Washington, DC, 1997.

NRMP, *1996 NRMP Data: 1996.* Washington, DC, 1996.

Slone R: Resident Selection. *Inv Rad* 1991;26:390.

Taylor C et al: The process of resident selection: A view from the residency director's desk. *Obstet Gynecol* 1995;85:299.

# Getting Residency Information and Applications

**4**

## WHERE CAN I LEARN ABOUT RESIDENCY PROGRAMS?

Before you start the application process, you will need to acquire enough information about the available residency programs to make a list of programs that fit your needs. Fortunately, there is no scarcity of data about training programs (Table 4–1). In fact, you will have to be selective and efficient in your information gathering. For example, career advisers can provide broad perspectives on a number of different programs, including clinical training and research. On the other hand, junior faculty, fellows, and house staff can give you the nitty-gritty about training at an individual program based on their residency experience. There is no one source that will tell everything as it relates to your goals.

### Career Adviser

Your career adviser, whether a department chairperson or a junior faculty member, should be aware of the programs that best fit your personal and career goals. Your adviser should also be able to provide information not found in Fellowship and Residency Electronic Interactive Database Access System (FREIDA) to help you understand the "personality" of the program. For example, he or she should know whether the program currently has a department chair, what type of research is conducted at that institution, the academic and clinical foci of the program, and the program's overall reputation.

If you are in luck, or if your school has been a "pipeline" into a specific program, your adviser might also know recent graduates of your medical school in the program whom you can contact. You can also request copies of the Match results of the last three graduating classes from your medical school and make phone calls on your own.

**YOU WILL HAVE TO LOOK HIGH AND LOW TO OBTAIN A BALANCED PICTURE.**

| TABLE 4–1. Information resources for residency programs. | |
|---|---|
| **Source** | **Contribution** |
| Career adviser (department chairperson, clinical faculty) | To identify appropriate programs which to apply to and inform you of the current status of the program. |
| Dean of students | To help you choose between specialties, pick an adviser, and assess overall competitiveness. |
| Faculty and house staff | To provide perspective on training and residency life. |
| Fourth-year medical students | To summarize what's hot/what's not: tips and warnings for prospects in your specialty. |
| AMA Fellowship and Residency Interactive Database Access (AMA-FREIDA) website (http://www.ama-assn.org/freida) | To provide current contact information for your target programs as well as detailed statistics. |
| *Graduate Medical Education Directory* (The "Green Book") | To provide contacts for residency programs. Next best thing to FREIDA. |
| *NRMP Program Results: Listing of Filled and Unfilled Programs* (available on the NRMP website at http://nrmp.aamc.org/nrmp) | To list the programs that did not fill all their spots in the previous Match. |
| *Transitional Year Program Directory* (The "Purple Book") | To give detailed listings of transitional year programs. |
| Directories published by some specialties | To supplement or update information in FREIDA. |
| San Francisco Residency Match website (http://www.sfmatch.org) | To obtain detailed information on the match process for neurology, neurosurgery, ophthalmology, and otolaryngology programs. |
| American Urological Association (AUA) website (http://www.auanet.org) | To obtain detailed information on the match process for urology residency programs. |

THE DEAN OF STUDENTS IS OFTEN AN OVERLOOKED RESOURCE.

## Dean of Students

This may seem obvious, but it is surprising how many students will pass up the opportunity to make an appointment, perhaps fearing that the dean is "too busy" to speak with them or is absorbed with weightier matters. Don't hesitate to schedule an appointment; this faculty person can be an excellent resource of information, advice, and advocacy.

Even a brief meeting can provide inside information about the workings of the Match at your school, advance word on how and when the dean's letter will be written, an early assessment of your academic progress as it might influence your specialty and program choice, and suggestions about who the "hot" advisers are. It is never too early to get some hints about strategies, both academic and personal. And remember, many a dean of students have gone through this process themselves, and often in the not too distant past.

## Faculty and House Staff

Faculty in your desired specialty that you meet on your junior and senior clerkships can complement information provided by your career adviser. Talk to as many of these people as possible and understand their perspectives (eg, geographic, academic vs clinical, etc). Senior residents can share their sense of the job market and their own job-hunting experiences. In addition, junior faculty and fellows can shed light on the residency programs that trained them. House staff can also provide information on programs they knew as medical students. Although house staff are in the best position to describe training and life as a resident, their perspective is limited to their own program and does not necessarily apply to any others.

## Senior Medical Students

After surviving their interviews and Match Day, graduating seniors are your best bet for practical application and interviewing tips. Debriefing some of these survivors will give you an additional "feel" for the application process and alert you to potential trouble spots. Most medical schools organize question-and-answer sessions with graduating seniors. Remember, though, that while the seniors have considerable "trench" experience, their perspectives are understandably limited when it comes to what programs might be best for you.

## Fellowship and Residency Electronic Interactive Database Access (AMA-FREIDA)

AMA-FREIDA (http://www.ama-assn.org/freida) is an annually updated PC-based database of residency programs, produced by the American Medical Association (AMA). It contains information on approximately 7,500 graduate medical programs and combined programs that are accredited by the Accreditation Council for Graduate Medical Education (ACGME). It is very easy to use and has supplanted the Graduate Medical Education Directory (aka the "Green Book") as the most popular source on residency programs. The data comes from the AMA Annual Survey of Graduate Medical Education Programs. These surveys are filled out in the fall and the data is entered in both October and February. In addition, programs can change some of the basic information throughout the year. Accessed through the Internet, FREIDA can search for programs by specialty, region or state, and program size, dividing an overwhelming amount of information on each program into eight manageable categories (Table 4–2). Included in each program's basic information is the name, address, phone number, and e-mail address of the program director and contact person and also the program's website address, which are very useful for obtaining answers to questions that are not answered on FREIDA. Each program has a 10-digit identifying number which will be listed in both the "Search Results" page and also under the program's basic information. Writing down these numbers will enable you to bypass the search engine and go directly to that specific program's information in the future.

FREIDA also has two other categories. Specialty Statistics provides general information on specialties and subspecialties, such as work hours, work environment, and average salary. Physician Workforce Information provides statistics given by residents and practicing physicians on finding employment,

> FREIDA IS A SELF-REPORTING DATABASE; IT DOES NOT COMPARE OR EVALUATE PROGRAMS.

---

**TABLE 4–2. Information in FREIDA.**

General program information
Educational environment
Work environment
Compensation and benefits
Clinical environment
Patient population
Medical benefits/institution features
Specialties in institution

---

| TABLE 4–3. Information in "Green Book" program listing. |
| --- |
| Program director's name, address, telephone number |
| Sponsoring institution |
| Other institutions with a major role in training |
| Number of training years |
| Total number of positions in program |
| Program ID number |

workplace environment, job satisfaction, etc. There are a few things to remember about FREIDA. The information is often incomplete or outdated. Moreover, all information is provided by the programs themselves without being verified. Sometimes program directors choose not to answer certain questions that they feel are irrelevant or embarrassing. Some programs do not fill out questionnaires at all and are listed only by name. Lastly, keep in mind that as a self-reporting database, FREIDA does not evaluate or compare programs.

## Roadmap to the Match Resource Center and Interview Insight™ on Medschool.com

The Roadmap to the Match Resource Center on Medschool.com's Community homepage (http://students.medschool.com) provides students with tips for the match at every step of the process. This resource center provides information for students on everything from choosing a specialty and writing a personal statement to applications and interviewing, and also has an updated Match calendar. The strongest areas of this resource center include the sections on application help and interview tips. Also unique to the Medschool.com website is a feature called Interview Insight™. Here students who have already interviewed at programs across the country have posted their thoughts on specific programs. For example, you can find out what each student felt were strengths and weaknesses about a particular program in pediatrics. Students can also leave tips for specific interviews and questions you should remember to ask while at your interview. Note that this is one of the few sources of student submitted feedback regarding residency programs in terms of reputation, workload, resident satisfaction, perks, and more. In addition to all this, the Medschool.com website provides moderated discussion forums for all major specialties as well as specific Match discussion forums with frequently asked questions.

## Graduate Medical Education Directory: The "Green Book"

The *Graduate Medical Education Directory* is an annually updated catalog of all training programs recognized by the Accreditation Council for Graduate Medical Education (ACGME). Despite its heft, the directory has very little information for each program other than the contact address and telephone number (Table 4–3).

The Green Book can be obtained at your office of student affairs or medical library. You can order your own copy by contacting:

American Medical Association
Order Department OP416795
PO Box 7046
Dover, DE 19903-7046
(800) 621-8335

THE "GREEN BOOK" IS BIG,
BUT IT'S NO FREIDA.

If you are an IMG with no convenient access to AMA-FREIDA, you should probably purchase your own copy of the Green Book. Although the program information contained in it is not as extensive as that in FREIDA, the Green Book does feature **some** facts not covered in FREIDA. These include visa and certification guidelines for foreign-born medical graduates seeking graduate medical education in the United States, detailed ACGME requirements for program accreditation by specialty, and state licensure requirements.

## Transitional Year Program Directory: The "Purple Book"

The Purple Book lists most transitional year programs and includes contact information, information on required and elective rotations, call schedule, etc. Because much of the same data is available on AMA-FREIDA, use the Purple Book as a secondary resource. It should be available at your office of student affairs and is also available over the Internet (http://www.ahme.med.edu). A copy can be ordered by calling or writing:

Association for Hospital Medical Education
1200 19th Street NW, Suite 300
Washington, DC 20036-2422
(202) 857-1196

## NRMP Program Results: Listing of Filled and Unfilled Programs

As described in Chapter 2, the *NRMP Program Results* lists all programs that did not fill their spots in the NRMP Match. If you are a weak candidate in a strong field, however, you might take a closer look at these programs. If not available at your student affairs office, the book can be ordered by calling or writing:

ATTN: Membership and Publication Orders
National Residency Matching Program
2450 N Street NW
Washington, DC 20037-1129
(202) 828-0416

## Specialty-Specific Directories

Several specialty organization websites maintain directories of training programs with contact information. A handful of directories (including those from family practice, internal medicine, psychiatry, physical medicine and rehabilitation, and preventive medicine) rival or surpass FREIDA in terms of comprehensiveness and appropriateness of information. In general, though, the specialty directories are not updated as frequently as FREIDA or the Green Book. See Chapter 3 for a list of specialty organization website addresses and contact information.

## Early Match Websites

For information on neurology, neurosurgery, ophthalmology, and otolaryngology programs, go to the San Francisco Residency Matching website at http://www.sfmatch.org. Information on urology programs can be found in the "Students and Residents" section at the American Urological Association website (http://www.auanet.org).

BE WARY OF PROGRAMS WITH UNFILLED SPOTS IN COMPETITIVE SPECIALTIES.

## HOW MANY PROGRAMS SHOULD I APPLY TO?

Most students want enough applications to ensure a healthy number of interviews, which in turn helps to ensure a successful match. The number of programs you apply to depends on a number of factors, namely: (1) your competitive standing; (2) the competitiveness of the specialty; (3) the competitiveness of the programs to which you are applying; and (4) whether you're participating in the couples match.

Because several factors figure into the equation, it's best to settle on a number with the help of your career adviser. If, however, you are even mildly interested in a particular program, write or call for an information packet (and application, if it is a non-ERAS residency program). If you remain unsure, err on the side of submitting too many applications (Figure 4–1). Don't worry about going overboard at this point. It is better to decline interview invitations later, rather than to realize that you do not have enough interviews to ensure a good match.

Consider the "Rule of Thirds" to achieve a balanced set of applications and minimize your chances of not matching. A third of your applications should go to your "dream programs" regardless of their competitiveness. Another third should include desirable programs where you have a solid chance of matching. The last third consists of acceptable programs that can serve as back ups. The Rule of Thirds works best in the less competitive specialties. Because of the recent implementation of ERAS and the ease of sending out applications, residency programs are receiving a higher volume of applications as compared to previous years. See "Your Specialty and the Match" (Chapter 3) to find the general prescription for the healthy number of applications in each field.

## HOW DO I OBTAIN APPLICATIONS?

The widespread use of ERAS by most specialties has greatly simplified this process. ERAS application materials are generally available after June 30th. Through ERAS, you will complete one common application that can be modified in terms of which letters of recommendation or personal statement you wish to be included for each residency program you apply to.

For those specialties that do not use ERAS, use FREIDA or the Green Book to contact programs for applications. This is the step that triggers an

**BETTER TO HAVE TOO MANY APPLICATIONS THAN TOO FEW.**

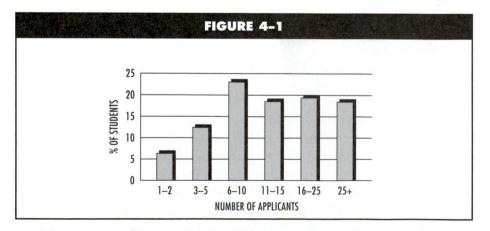

### FIGURE 4–1

Number of residency applications made by U.S. fourth-year medical students.

avalanche of paperwork. To keep yourself sane (and stable) during this process, **follow two rules from the start:** (1) Finalize your list of target programs before beginning the application process. Adding and dropping applications in midstream will mean having to track that much more paperwork; (2) Try to complete each step of each application at the same time. For example, request at once all required transcripts.

To request applications, purchase pre-stamped postcards at the post office. If you're using a computer word processor, it's simple and worth the effort to create three sets of labels. On the first set, write a brief note requesting information and an application. Type your address on the second set, and the name of the program director and the program addresses on the third set of labels. Then, simply attach the three labels to the face of the postcard in the appropriate spots (Figure 4–2).

You should send for applications and program information **no later than early August.** Allow two to three weeks to receive applications from programs, then follow up with phone calls as needed. If you fall behind time on requests, consider calling all the programs directly for information and applications. It's worth the cost of the phone calls and you might be able to get answers to some simple questions while requesting applications.

## WHAT SHOULD I BE LOOKING FOR IN A PROGRAM?

Before you set up your list of programs to apply to, you need to have some idea of your priorities. You don't need crystal-ball clarity at this point, but it is necessary for you to think through the following issues rather early in the process. You should review the following issues when you start interviewing.

### Location

Location is a critical though highly personal issue. Some candidates are restricted by employment requirements of their significant other. Others want

### FIGURE 4-2

Dear Program Director,
Please send me information and an application for your residency program in General Surgery to the address below. Thank you.

USA

Your brief message

John Carter
911 Honors Ave.
Chicago, IL 12345

Michael Crichton, MD
Department of Surgery
Jurassic School of Medicine
111 Cretaceous Blvd., S-1234
Mesozoic City, CA 12345

FREIDA generated label

Your address label

Sample application request postcard.

| **TABLE 4-4. Some application hot spots.** |
| --- |
| Boston |
| Chicago |
| Hawaii |
| San Diego |
| San Francisco |
| Seattle |

to be near family, or wish to use residency as an opportunity to establish contacts in the community in which ultimately they hope to practice. If you are adventurous and have no serious "attachments," then consider programs that will place you on new terrain. Many doing preliminary or transitional PGY-1 years take advantage of the chance to experience another city with limited commitment. It might be your last chance to do so before marital and family responsibilities catch up with you. In either case, recognize that even weak programs can be competitive if they have an attractive location (Table 4-4).

Most students acquire a sense of regional variations in styles and attitudes towards residency training. For example, many students who have trained on both coasts report that faculty tend to be less formal in the West Coast institutions. In the course of your interviews, you may pick up some regional flavors in the medical training available. Decide what suits your tastes.

## Setting

Most applicants' career plans can be categorized as either academically oriented, clinically oriented, or both. You want to find a program that fits your preference. Many programs can be classified into the following settings: university, community, or urban/county. Many of these programs run services at more than one hospital, thus offering their residents exposure to multiple settings. It's worth your while to ask about the amount of time you would spend at each hospital.

**University:** A university medical school affiliation is advantageous for two reasons: (1) medical schools offer teaching opportunities; and (2) the presence of medical students ensures a setting geared towards teaching the residents as well. Teaching conferences are generally of higher quality in university programs than in other settings. There are, however, a few drawbacks. For starters, university programs can be more intense, which tends to contribute to a lower level of sociability among the residents. Residents in university programs tend to have greater access to knowledgeable consultants, but some residents complain that because of this wealth of specialists and consultants they have less autonomy and decision-making responsibility. Likewise, for better or worse, patient populations in a university setting are often not representative of what the resident will encounter in community practice after training. The plus is that university programs tend to be based in tertiary care centers that give their residents exposure to the more unusual or interesting cases.

**Community:** Residents usually receive kinder, gentler training at a community program. Salaries and benefits also tend to be more humane. Because there is less academic pressure, residents are typically more relaxed and have more time for reading. However, well-organized rounds and conferences may be lacking. Like urban and county programs, community programs are academically less prestigious. Given the large proportion of private patients and private attendings, you may not receive the same degree of patient responsibility or experience with certain procedures.

**Urban/county:** If you really want hands-on experience, city and county hospitals will virtually give you blisters. You can forget academic theorization here; you'll be taught to manage a large patient volume: a population largely consisting of urban poor. Most likely, you will be heavily involved in the decision-making process and will gain more experience with a variety of invasive procedures. Unfortunately, at a county or city hospital you are frequently overworked and underpaid. These programs often lack the academic prestige and name-recognition of their university equivalents, with notable exceptions such as Massachusetts General Hospital. In addition, ancillary support tends to be weaker, and formal teaching is often uneven and disorganized.

## Stability

With graduate medical education facing drastic cuts in federal funding, you should determine how financially secure a residency program is. How much of its funding comes from federal sources? How well off is the parent hospital or university?

In addition, many teaching hospitals (especially on the East and West Coasts) are now experiencing unprecedented competition from managed care. Does the parent hospital enjoy a robust patient base, or is it floundering in a rising tide of managed care?

## Reputation

A program's reputation invariably comes into play if the applicant is considering fellowship training or a career in academic medicine. Its reputation, whether deserved or not, can visibly influence your ability to secure competitive fellowships or faculty appointments in the future. However, if the program is too large, no matter how prestigious, you may have to sweat to get the strong personal recommendations necessary to secure a competitive fellowship. The reality in community practice is that most patients will not know or really care what medical school you graduated from, much less where you trained.

## Subspecialty Strengths

If you're considering subspecialty training after residency, you might reevaluate programs with strengths in that subspecialty. In addition, it never hurts to have a well-known "name" in a subspecialty write you a strong letter of recommendation.

## Educational Environment

Because residency programs are a form of post-graduate education, you need to appraise the educational philosophy and facilities at the institutions that interest you. Pay attention to the following aspects of residency programs:

**Curriculum/conferences:** Residents depend on well-organized conferences and teaching rounds to expand their knowledge base and reinforce what they already know. Most programs have, or are developing, an organized required curriculum that exposes residents to all major topics in the specialty during their training. The curriculum might include rotations, conferences, and syllabi with assigned reading. In some specialties, there is a lot of variation in emphasis and formality; **you** have to decide which combination best fits your needs. For example, some family practice programs emphasize obstetrics; others practically exclude it. Some medicine programs feature heavy experience and training in HIV; others have next to none.

**Faculty teaching:** The teaching that residents receive from faculty, and the rapports they establish with them can be correlated to a number of factors: faculty-to-resident ratio, program setting, proportion of private attendings, and overall size of the program. A large program cannot provide as much personal mentoring, but thankfully you are less at the mercy of a few quirky personalities. When you visit the program, get a sense of what interest the faculty maintains in the training and welfare of its house staff. What type of feedback does the house staff receive from the faculty? Is there a mechanism for evaluation of the faculty?

**Research and teaching opportunities:** While research and teaching opportunities are nearly essential for those planning on an academic career or subspecialty training, they are also desirable even if you have no plans of staying within academic walls. When you assess the research opportunities at a program, ask yourself the following questions. Are there well-established researchers available to guide residents? Is there time allotted for research, either as a requirement or as an elective? How successful is the program in securing grants, hospital funding or internal funding for research? How satisfied are the residents who are presently completing their projects? Or, for that matter, how many dissatisfied residents will cite a lack of institutional financial support?

## Work Environment

Don't forget to survey the working environment when you size up a residency program. After all, you'll be putting in a lot of hours in that set of buildings with their cast of characters. So don't overlook these considerations:

**Work versus education:** Many programs are guilty of exploiting the "cheap labor" of residents without providing a rich educational experience. Residency is "learning by doing" to be sure, but be on the lookout for how service versus education is balanced.

**Patient population/load:** The optimal patient load will provide you with enough clinical experience and will leave you with adequate time and energy to read and attend teaching conferences. Patient load is often a function of the program's setting (see above). On your interview visits, ask for an average patient census, and discreetly ask residents how they feel about the workload. Know what medical problems are common in the population served by the program. For example, an orthopedics program may get more than its share of trauma cases because of its location near several major highways. In addition, you want to get a feel for other characteristics of the patient population, such as ethnicity/language (a large Spanish-speaking population?), socioeconomic status (urban poor?), and attitude (typical Saturday night ER crowd?). Keep in mind that the best training environment does not have to match that of your future practice.

**Patient responsibilities:** The whole point of residency training is to provide you with the experience and skills necessary for you to practice medicine unsupervised. When you visit the program, find out if the attending allows the resident to "run the show," or if the resident needs approval for major decisions. Next, is backup assistance readily available if the resident or intern needs help? Or are you on your own even if World War III breaks out on your shift or call night?

ONE SURGICAL RESIDENT TO ANOTHER. . . .
Q: WHAT'S WRONG WITH EVERY-OTHER-NIGHT CALL?
A: YOU MISS OUT ON HALF OF THE CASES.

**Call schedule:** Call schedules vary widely by specialty, setting, year of training, and training site (for programs with multiple sites). Recognize the range of calls that can deprive you of a good night's sleep (Table 4–5). The house officer will often encounter a mix of calls during the year. How much sleep you typically get during a call night and how late you work post-call is almost as important as how often you're on call. For many specialties, call frequency often varies by training year.

Closely, tied to call schedule is the number of work hours per week. Information is available on the FREIDA website (http://www.ama-assn.org/freida) and Medschool.com (http://www.medschool.com) under "Specialty Profiles." Know your own threshold and the workload you are willing to tolerate.

**Ancillary support:** No one is an island, and your team certainly doesn't go it alone in caring for your patients. Good nursing support, consulting services, phlebotomy, laboratory, hospital information services, transport services, and emergency room care are keys to a smooth clinical work experience. As an intern, you will often be used as a person of last resort to fill any gaps in ancillary support (unless you scut the poor medical student).

*Esprit de corps:* *Esprit de corps* is a familiar, albeit foreign, term for morale. Trust your intuition as well as your powers of observation. Are the residents "happy campers"? Is the atmosphere friendly or competitive? What kind of camaraderie exists among the residents? Among faculty, house staff, and administration? Look for the answers on your visit by asking the house staff and ancillary staff. Quietly divide and conquer. It is usually easier to get an honest answer in private from a departing resident than the chief resident or the program director in front of 20 other interviewees. Afterwards, assess the quality of your own experience during the visit.

> **DON'T FORGET TO ASK HOW MUCH SLEEP YOU GET WHEN ON CALL AND ABOUT THE LENGTH OF THE POST-CALL DAY.**

> **WHAT RESIDENTS DO NOT SAY MAY BE MORE TELLING THAN WHAT THEY DO SAY.**

| | TABLE 4–5. Types of calls. | |
|---|---|---|
| **Type** | **Description** | **Ask About** |
| Long call | House officer admits patients throughout a 24-hour period. Sometimes there is a nightfloat that takes admissions after a certain hour and cross-cover that assists a team if a member has clinic that day. | How many admissions per night, how much sleep intern/resident typically gets, and whether there is a nightfloat or cross-cover. |
| Short call | House officer takes admissions from morning until a certain hour at night. | When short call ends and if there is an admissions cap. |
| Home/beeper call | House officer is on call outside hospital. How often the resident comes into the hospital depends on nature of admission or issue of current patient; and if other members of the team are in hospital. | How often does the intern/resident come into the hospital. |
| Jeopardy call | House officer can be placed on call on short notice to cover for sick colleague or to alleviate heavy patient admissions. Usually used on otherwise light or no call rotations. | How often does the intern/resident come into the hospital. |
| Nightfloat | House officer on a dedicated night rotation takes admissions for on-call team after a certain time (i.e., midnight). Admissions are transferred to another team in the morning. | How many weeks are you on nightfloat, and at what time nightfloat duties start. |

## Salary

Residents are paid so little that salary is usually not the central issue. Interestingly enough, most of your paycheck comes from the federal government rather than the program itself: thus, you may be fattening the bottom line of a hospital that is not even paying you. The average income of an intern in 1999–2000 was $34,985. Don't bother calculating your pay per hour; it will only depress you. Salary information is readily available on FREIDA. Your income usually rises incrementally during your residency training, but not by much. It is critical to factor in cost of living when comparing salaries: $30,000 will take you much further in Louisville, Kentucky, than $32,000 in Los Angeles (Table 4–6).

For many, these low figures are reason enough to moonlight. Once licensed to practice medicine (typically, after the first year), you can usually earn anywhere from $20 to $120 per hour working in a variety of settings, including emergency rooms, nursing homes, outpatient clinics (ie, "doc in the box"); doing insurance company physical exams; and even working in prisons. Some programs actually provide in-house moonlighting opportunities, which can be a major source of supplementary income. In-house jobs will often take into account your regular call schedule, making it easier to moonlight during residency. On the other hand, many programs officially ban moonlighting or actively discourage it, so tactfully ask about it on your visit, and someone (usually a graduating resident) will give you the scoop.

**IN-HOUSE MOONLIGHTING OFFERS THE BEST OF BOTH WORLDS.**

## Benefits

Though everyone remembers salary, don't forget about other benefits. Many programs offer medical insurance, dental services, paid drug prescriptions, employee health services, and psychiatric counseling (Table 4–7). Shop around carefully, especially if you have a family. Be aware that certain benefits at some programs are only available if the resident pays a portion of the cost. You don't want to end up spending part of your meager salary for benefits that other programs would have provided for free. When evaluating insurance, ask yourself: (1) who is covered (ie, family); (2) what is covered; (3) what costs do I pay out of pocket?

In addition to health benefits, you want to ensure that your program offers adequate life, disability, and liability insurance. After four years in medical school and untold thousands of dollars, you (and your family) don't want to be left high and dry if you get sick, have an accident, or something else goes wrong. If you're planning on starting a family during residency training, then scrutinize the rules on maternity/paternity leave (Table 4–8). Find out if the policy is writ-

**KEY BENEFITS = $$$**

| TABLE 4–6. Average 1999 Resident stipends. | | | | | |
|---|---|---|---|---|---|
| Year | All | Northeast | South | Midwest | West |
| PGY-1 | $34,985 | $36,928 | $33,887 | $34,908 | $33,273 |
| PGY-2 | 36,564 | 38,723 | 35,001 | 36,192 | 36,133 |
| PGY-3 | 38,214 | 40,660 | 36,336 | 37,493 | 38,663 |
| PGY-4 | 39,847 | 42,413 | 37,789 | 38,785 | 41,094 |
| PGY-5 | 41,424 | 44,164 | 39,133 | 40,116 | 43,403 |
| PGY-6 | 43,045 | 46,086 | 40,581 | 41,541 | 45,199 |

**TABLE 4–7. Survey of health benefits offered by residency programs.**

| Benefit | % Fully Paid (Resident/ Family) | % Offered/Cost Shared (Resident/Family) | % Offered/Not Paid (Resident/Family) | % Not Available (Resident/ Family) |
|---|---|---|---|---|
| Group medical insurance | 59/42 | 40/53 | 0/6 | 1/1 |
| Group dental insurance | 47/34 | 33/40 | 13/18 | 7/8 |
| Vision | 34/27 | 28/35 | 8/9 | 31/28 |
| Drug prescriptions | 52/42 | 42/50 | 2/3 | 4/5 |
| Psychiatric benefits | 59/47 | 37/44 | 1/5 | 2/4 |
| Counseling | 59/49 | 34/38 | 2/4 | 6/9 |

ten or if it varies with each case (and personality). Of course, to date maternity leave policies tend to be more generous than paternity leave policies.

Other benefits to consider include parking, housing, meals, vacation, education leave for conferences, library services (eg, photocopying), and child care (Table 4–9).

## HOW DO I ORGANIZE THIS INFORMATION?

Great. You know what to look for. But now you need to be able to organize and evaluate all the data. You are already receiving information from multiple sources: FREIDA, your adviser, and house officers at your medical institution. You will be flooded with more information on your visits to the programs. We've included a Program Evaluation Worksheet (PEW) which will allow you to organize information conveniently and evaluate a program objectively (Figures 4–3A and 4–3B). Make a copy for each program on your application hit list. Take them with you on the interview trail to record notes and impressions.

## REFERENCES

AMA Fellowship and Residency Interactive Database Access (AMA-FREIDA) website (http://www.ama-assn.org/freida).
American Urological Association (AUA) website (http://www.auanet.org).

**TABLE 4–8. Issues addressed by a complete parental leave policy.**

Duration of leaves allowed before and after delivery

Which category of leave credited

Whether leave is paid or unpaid

Whether provision is made for continuation of insurance benefits and the payment of premiums

Whether sick leave and vacation time may be accrued from year to year or used in advance

Whether make-up time will be paid

Policies for adoption

Whether schedule accommodations are allowed

## TABLE 4–9. Survey of non-health benefits offered by residency programs.

| Benefit | % Fully Paid | % Offered/ Cost Shared | % Offered/ Not Paid | % Not Available |
|---|---|---|---|---|
| Life insurance | 82 | 11 | 3 | 5 |
| Disability insurance | 77 | 5 | 6 | 13 |
| Housing | 53 | 11 | 14 | 71 |
| Parking | 61 | 15 | 20 | 4 |
| Meals at work | 23 | 28 | 24 | 26 |
| Meals while on call | 84 | 11 | 1 | 4 |

## FIGURE 4–3A

Program Name _____

Date of Visit _____

| Factor | Comments |
|---|---|
| Location | |
| Setting | |
| Reputation | |
| Stability of program | |
| Subspecialty strengths | |
| **Education** | |
| Conferences/rounds | |
| Faculty teaching | |
| Post-residency plans of graduates | |
| Research/teaching opportunities | |
| **Work Environment** | |
| Patient population/load | |
| Patient responsibilities | |
| Call frequency/ hours per week | |
| Ancillary support (eg, nursing) | |
| On call support (eg, nightfloat, admission caps) | |
| Health benefits | |
| Non-health benefits | |
| Vacation/sick leave/ parenting leave | |

Program Evaluation Worksheet (PEW).

**FIGURE 4-3B**

**Other Factors/Notes**

Gut feeling

| Advantages | Disadvantages |
|---|---|
| | |

**Preliminary Rank**

☐ Top third ☐ Middle third ☐ Bottom third ☐ Do not rank

**Interview Log**

| Name/Address | Notes |
|---|---|
| | |
| | |
| | |

Association of American Medical Colleges: COTH *Survey of House Staff Stipends, Benefits and Funding, 1994*. Washington, DC, 1994.

Association of American Medical Colleges: COTH *Survey of House Staff Stipends, Benefits and Funding, 1999*. Washington, DC, 1999.

Bickel J: Maternity leave policies for residents: An overview of issues and problems. *Acad Med* 1989;64:498.

Medschool.com website (http://www.medschool.com).

Reiss G: A guide to obtaining postgraduate medical training. *Resident & Staff Physician* 1982; p. 111.

San Francisco Residency Match website (http://www.sfmatch.org).

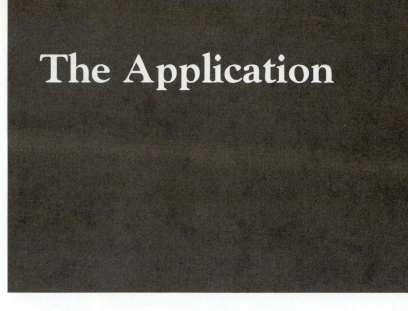

# The Application

## WHAT IS IN AN APPLICATION?

There are three categories that most applicants will be applying to: early match specialties (neurosurgery, neurology, ophthalmology, ENT, urology), non-ERAS specialties (currently only radiation oncology and plastic surgery), and ERAS specialties. For the latter two categories, brochures and applications (for non-ERAS specialties only) from the programs of your choice should start pouring in by early August. If you are participating in early match, you will need to start this process sooner. For all specialties, a complete program application file consists of several documents or sets of documents that you must assemble, track, and finally send off. You will be pulling together its components all summer and into early fall (Table 5–1). If you don't already own a file drawer or document storage box, buy a set of hanging file folders or an accordion file, and a set of manila file folders to organize your materials.

## HOW DO I ORGANIZE THE PAPERWORK?

For ERAS specialties and for many early match specialties, you will fill out one common application. However, for non-ERAS specialties, you will notice that each program has its own set of application requirements. These requirements are outlined in the program's cover letter, or within the application itself. Some will ask you to complete the NRMP Universal Application; others will include their own forms. Some programs want your undergraduate transcript in addition to your medical school transcript. To help you keep track of who wants what, photocopy enough copies of the enclosed Worksheet for Application Requirements  (WAR) to list all the programs that you are applying to (Figure 5–1).

Remember that in order to keep paperwork from escalating out of control: (1) do not add any new programs to your list after you have started work on the applications; and (2) try to complete one item (eg, transcript obtaining) for all applications at the same time.

FOR MAXIMUM EFFICIENCY AND MINIMUM CONFUSION, ORGANIZE APPLICATION REQUIREMENTS ON A WORKSHEET (LIKE OURS).

| TABLE 5-1. Common elements of an application file. | | |
|---|---|---|
| **Document** | **Function** | **Quick Advice** |
| Program application | Foundation of application file | Request by early August. Better to get too many than too few. |
| Dean's letter | Compendium of written evaluations compiled by Dean of Student Affairs | Take an active role in helping dean by editing/supplementing content if possible. Clarify any inaccuracies. |
| Letters of recommendation | Written testimonials from faculty familiar with your work | Solicit letters no later than August. Confirm that writer feels comfortable writing a "strong" letter. |
| Transcript | Academic record | Proofread an unofficial copy before having them sent out. |
| CV | Summary of your credentials, activities and accomplishments | Pull together by July. Nice to have for personal statement and to accompany requests for letters of recommendation. |
| Personal statement | Opportunity to establish your own voice and distinguish yourself from other applicants | Finish personal statement before applications arrive. Multiple reviewers and revisions are key. |

## WHO EVALUATES MY APPLICATION?

**THE BUSIER THE SELECTION COMMITTEE, THE MORE LITTLE THINGS WILL BOTHER THEM.**

**THE PROGRAM SECRETARY CAN BE A POWERFUL ALLY.**

As you assemble your application materials, remember your audience. The residency selection committee is usually composed of the residency director, several faculty members, and a few house officers. They are **extremely busy people**, and would rather be doing something other than screening your application on a Saturday afternoon. Make their job as pleasant as possible by having a neat, professional-looking application with clear, succinct answers.

Remember that in addition to the faculty, departmental or administrative assistants can make or break an application. The comments they provide the committee on their interactions with you may well color the committee's initial impressions. If the departmental secretary likes you well enough, he or she may actually push for your application or direct it to a receptive committee member. If you miss any deadlines, friendly administrative assistants may bend rules to keep your application in the running. If anything goes wrong in your application, you will need every ally you can get.

## HOW DO THEY EVALUATE MY APPLICATION?

Once your application arrives on the desk of the program director, he or she will direct its contents to a number of different readers at different phases in the evaluation process. The typical process can be divided into several stages, which we will outline for you.

### Screening

In the initial phase of the evaluation process, your application is usually screened by a select few overworked committee members after hours during the week or during weekend afternoons. Screeners will read your application, the letters of recommendation, selected portions of the dean's letter, and the transcript. When they look at the dean's letter, committee members typically focus on junior and senior clerkship evaluations in their field, and

**FIGURE 5-1**

**Directions:** Fill in blanks below with requested numbers/names/dates. Under **Application Requirements**, list each requirement by name. Once you have assembled the item for that application, check it off.

| Program Name | Application Mailing Address | Contact & Phone # | App. Deadline | Application Requirements | Notes |
|---|---|---|---|---|---|
| | | | | ☐ ☐ ☐ ☐ ☐ | |
| | | | | ☐ ☐ ☐ ☐ ☐ | |
| | | | | ☐ ☐ ☐ ☐ ☐ | |
| | | | | ☐ ☐ ☐ ☐ ☐ | |
| | | | | ☐ ☐ ☐ ☐ ☐ | |

Worksheet for application requirements.

scan the summary paragraph for the crucial code words (See Table 5–4). Note that the personal statement tends to carry little or no weight at this point in the process, since the screener has another 50 files or so to plow through. The screener then completes an evaluation form, which will toss your application into one of three piles: a recommendation to interview, maybe interview, or not interview. Some programs grant interviews on a rolling basis, so again it's best to get your application in as early as possible.

## The Interview

Many conscientious interviewers will review your file before the actual interview. Others will prefer to review the file while you're sitting there in their office, which can be distracting to you when you're already under stress. Busy interviewers zoom in on areas that consistently give the most information bang for the buck, like the CV, transcript, letters of recommendation from "known" writers, and the dean's letter. The importance of your personal statement will depend on the individual interviewer and the specialty.

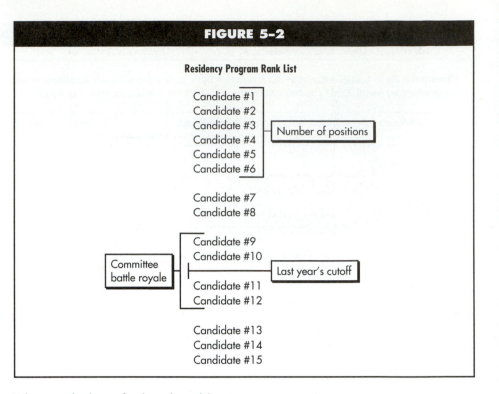

**FIGURE 5-2**

Residency Program Rank List

Candidate #1
Candidate #2
Candidate #3 ⎤ Number of positions
Candidate #4
Candidate #5
Candidate #6

Candidate #7
Candidate #8

Candidate #9
Candidate #10
Committee battle royale — Last year's cutoff
Candidate #11
Candidate #12

Candidate #13
Candidate #14
Candidate #15

Where most battles are fought on the rank list.

## Ranking Sessions

After all the interviews have been completed, there is at least one highly charged, exhausting session in which the full committee attempts to rank the candidates they've seen. In many cases, not all applicants interviewed are ranked. The real committee battles are **not** fought over the names high on the rank list. The top applicants are easy to rank. Rather, the committee members will squabble over the names in the middle ground. As you might expect, the battle heats up near the rank spot to which they had to drop last year to fill their program (if they filled at all) (Figure 5–2).

As the meeting wears on, the application files are usually subjected to closer scrutiny. At this point, the committee is likely to overanalyze your personal statement. Anything unusual in your personal statement (e.g., a description of the grunge band that you hope to organize during your residency) or the rest of your application is much more likely to be judged bizarre than as a factor weighted in your favor. Bottom line: be smart, assertive, yet conservative in tone and approach—that is, don't take unnecessary chances.

## Selection Factors

Throughout the evaluation process, the selection committee tests its pool of applicants against certain criteria important to its program. You may think that all programs want is an applicant elected to AΩA, spectacular board scores, and "Honors" plastered all over the transcript. However, academic standing is only part of the story. What good is stellar academic performance if the applicant does not interact smoothly with current faculty, house staff and administration? Program directors want residents who work hard and perform well as part of a team. According to the program directors themselves, the factors most important to residency committees tend to be personal (Table 5–2).

**TABLE 5-2. Factors most important to program directors.**

1. Attitude
2. Stability
3. Interpersonal skills
4. Academic performance
5. Maturity

THE APPLICATION

92

**FIGURE 5-3**

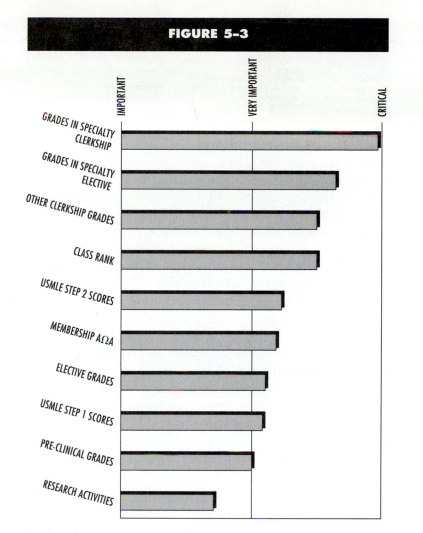

Academic factors important to residency directors.

Of course, overall academic performance is still important. Among the major academic selection factors, grades in the specialty rotation and electives seem to be the most crucial (Figure 5–3). Bear in mind that the significance of these academic factors varies from specialty to specialty. For example, psychiatry residency directors rate AΩA membership as "somewhat important," whereas general surgery residency directors consider this honor as a "very important" academic selection factor. See Chapter 3, "Your Specialty and the Match," to find out the key criteria in your specialty.

# PROGRAM APPLICATIONS

## ERAS Applications

Developed by the Association of American Medical Colleges (AAMC), the Electronic Residency Application Service (ERAS) was first employed in 1995–96 and has four components utilizing the Internet: MyERAS applicant webstation, the Dean's Office Workstation, the Program Directors Workstation, and the ERAS PostOffice. Using MyERAS, applicants complete their applications, select residency programs, and attach any supporting documents. ERAS® 2001 has been updated so that applicants will no longer have to use computer diskettes to store and transfer their applications. Once completed, the application is transmitted to the Dean's Office Workstation, where the dean's letter, letters of recommendation, and transcripts are added to the application in a separate file. Your photo will be scanned and attached to the application as well. The completed application is then transmitted to the ERAS PostOffice, where it can be downloaded (except for the dean's letter, which is held in the ERAS PostOffice until November 1st) by the applicant's chosen residency programs via the Program Directors Workstation at any time.

With ERAS it is theoretically much easier to keep track of all the documents and forms in your application: you will know exactly what went to whom. The intuitive and user-friendly student software automatically guides you through a series of windows to create your application. It's so easy that many students do not even touch the instruction manual (Table 5–3). ERAS applications can be customized in two important ways: (1) You can individualize your personal statement for each program; and (2) you can decide which letters of recommendation go to which program, if you have a choice of letters. Because of the ERAS numbering system, programs will not know how many letters of recommendation you are requesting. Currently, you can send a maximum of four letters, not including the dean's letter, to any program. Both your program selection list and the total number of programs you are applying to are confidential information between you and the dean's office.

ERAS® 2001 will be used by most residency programs in anesthesiology, dermatology, diagnostic radiology, emergency medicine, family practice, general surgery, internal medicine, obstetrics and gynecology, orthopedic surgery, pathology, pediatrics, physical medicine and rehabilitation, psychiatry, transitional year programs, all Army and Navy GME-1 positions, and combined family practice-psychiatry, internal medicine-emergency medicine, internal medicine-family practice, internal medicine-pediatrics, internal medicine-psychiatry and internal medicine-physical medicine and rehabilitation programs. Application materials will be distributed after June 30, 2000. Be aware that some programs in the above specialties may not be using ERAS, so you may need to contact these programs separately for applications.

U.S. medical students, including osteopathic students, will receive their ERAS materials through their student affairs office.

Foreign medical school graduates interested in using ERAS should contact the Educational Commission for Foreign Medical Graduates (ECFMG). ECFMG acts as the dean's office for foreign graduates; it will attach dean's letters, transcripts, and letters of recommendation, and transmit USMLE scores.

ECFMG-ERAS Program
P.O. Box 13467
Philadelphia, PA 19101-3467
U.S.A.
http://www.ecfmg.org

**TABLE 5-3. Major steps in ERAS.**

Fill out common application form

Create a personal statement

Request letters of recommendation

Select residency programs to receive applications

Canadian medical school graduates interested in applying to U.S. residency programs should contact the Canadian Resident Matching Service:

Canadian Resident Matching Service
151 Slater St., Suite 802
Ottawa, Ontario K1P-5H3 Canada

Applicants can use ERAS on any computer (PC or Mac) with World Wide Web access and any Netscape, Internet Explorer, AOL or other compatible browser (version 4.0 or higher). Most medical schools have student computer workstations containing ERAS.

Once your application is transmitted to the Dean's Office Workstation, you cannot make any changes to your application or delete any programs. However, if you decide to apply to additional programs, you can modify your application for these programs before you send it to the dean's office. Be sure to check with the individual programs what their deadline for applications is. Applicants can check on their documents via the Applicant Document Tracking System (ADTS) 24 hours a day.

Current ERAS fees are as follows: For each specialty, the application plus up to 10 programs selected will cost $60. An additional $6 will be assessed for programs 11-20, $12 for programs 21-30, and $25 for programs >30. Foreign medical graduates will also be charged an additional fee from the ECFMG since it will serve as the dean's office.

Applicants are currently being charged a $45 fee for an unlimited number of USMLE/NBME transcripts (which include your Step 1 and Step 2 scores). Once your request reaches the ERAS PostOffice, the NBME will begin processing it within one week. Your Step 2 scores will not be sent automatically to residency programs unless you include a transcript request with your application, send an electronic request separate from the application, or mark the box on the application which automatically sends your updated transcript. ERAS does not transmit National Board of Osteopathic Medical Examiners (NBOME) transcripts or scores. If you wish to report these scores, contact the individual programs to find out how they should be submitted.

For more information go to http://www.aamc.org/~eras.

## Early Match Applications

Most early match applications (except urology, go to the American Urological Association website at http://www.auanet.org for more information) will be handled and processed by the Central Application Service (CAS), provided by the San Francisco Matching program. However, remember that while CAS is mandatory for ophthalmology and ENT programs, it is only mandatory for some programs in neurology and neurosurgery and optional for the others. CAS materials are sent to registered applicants generally by early July. The CAS process is similar to ERAS in that you fill out one common application. After obtaining one copy of each supporting document, mail the entire application packet to CAS. Overnight delivery is recommended so that you can track its receipt. The application will then be copied and sent to your selected programs. Application fees are currently $60 total for the first 10 programs. An additional $10 will be charged for programs 11–20, $15 for 21–30, $20 for 31–40, and $25 for >40. For more information, go to http://www.sfmatch.org.

MAKE SURE YOUR SCHOOL SENDS OUT YOUR ERAS APPLICATION IN A TIMELY MANNER.

DO NOT LET APPLICATION FEES DISCOURAGE YOU FROM SUBMITTING A COMFORTABLE NUMBER OF APPLICATIONS.

## Paper (non-ERAS) Applications

For non-ERAS programs, the NRMP Universal Application was created to simplify the application process. The idea was that you would complete this application only once, and then send photocopies of the application to programs that accept it. Unfortunately, programs that accept the Universal Application are in the minority. The majority of programs insist on using their own forms. The writing process can be very frustrating since these "custom" applications often differ only slightly from the Universal Application in content, but use unique layouts, forcing the applicant back to his or her typewriter/word processor for yet another round of cut-and-paste.

If any of your prospective programs request the Universal Application, **fill it out first**. Much of the material that it calls for will resurface in other application forms. Some students find it helpful to hire a secretarial service to handle the paperwork and produce top-quality customized application materials. If you are on busy clinical rotations, or don't have the skills or compulsiveness to track all the details yourself, these services can be a sanity preserver.

When you receive a program application, **make at least two photocopies**. Write the necessary information by hand neatly on one of the photocopies before typing on the original. If you mortally mess up the original and have no time to request another, the second photocopy serves as a backup. As you complete the applications, keep the following tips in mind:

> ► For information to be filled in on the form itself, use a good electric typewriter with perfect error correction. Or, if you are experienced and ambitious, use a word processor. This second method involves the risky process of feeding applications into laser printers or photocopiers (the overlay method)—a test of your alignment skills. Word processing is best reserved for the personal statement, where looks count and a nice, proportionally-spaced computer font is more compact and readable than most typewriter fonts. If you can't do it right, get help from a computer-savvy friend or a secretarial service.

> ► Avoid filling a blank on an application with "See CV" or "See Personal Statement." These abbreviations may make sense to you, but they can annoy residency directors to no end, since the personal statement or CV is often a loose piece of paper elsewhere in your application file. In addition, these shorthand terms bespeak a certain lack of motivation. You can, of course, abbreviate specific titles or similar terms in the information requested if necessary (eg, "U" for "University," "Schl" for "School," etc.) If the space provided is too small, fill it in with the most important information; **only then** add "Also see CV" or "Also see Personal Statement."

> ► When you are finished, **make and file a photocopy of the complete application**. Applications do get lost in the mail, and you might need to fax or send a replacement by express mail to the program if the post office fouls up. Also, having your copy handy right before your interview is a helpful memory refresher. Reviewing what you wrote in your application will help you anticipate questions and avoid possible inconsistencies between what you put down on paper and what you say in person.

If a program high on your list gives you the choice of the NRMP Universal Application or their own form, use their form and resist the urge to take the easy way out, especially if they indicate preference for their form.

GIVE THEM WHAT THEY ASK FOR
WHERE THEY WANT IT.

# THE DEAN'S LETTER

As we mentioned earlier, the letter from your dean is a key item at the screening and interview stages of the application process. Deans' letters convey a variety of different types of information about you to discerning committee members (Figure 5–4). Although the dean's letter is supposed to be an objective evaluation of your medical school performance, most deans' letters come across as enthusiastic letters of recommendation, thus bolstering many average or weaker applicants, but possibly diluting the very strong ones.

## FIGURE 5-4

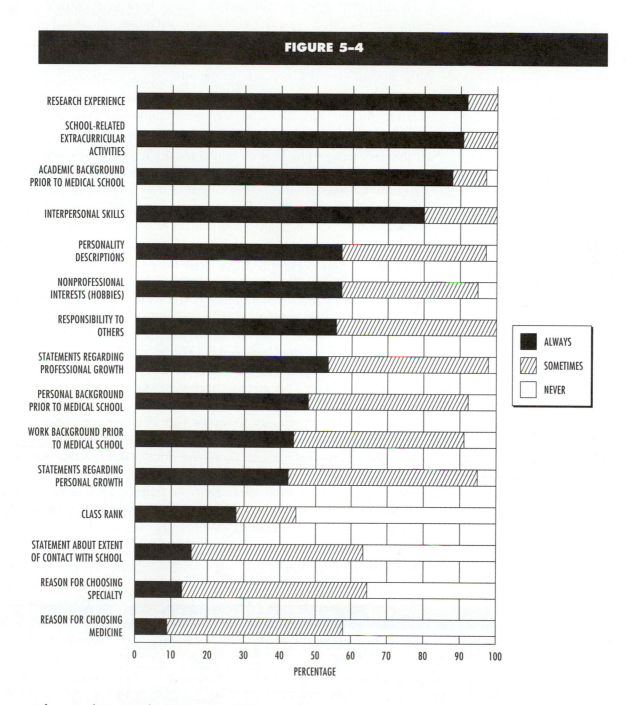

Information that commonly appears in deans' letters.

Though deans' letters can vary a lot, they typically contain the following components:

► **Personal background information.** This includes pertinent and noteworthy information from your undergraduate career and medical school application (eg, graduating *magna cum laude*, leadership positions, etc.).

► **Pre-clinical evaluations.** This section will tell the committee about your preclinical honors; or, on the other hand, about any irregularities in progress or required remediation.

► **Clinical evaluations.** Typically the longest portion of the dean's letter. The majority of letters will include quotes from your clinical evaluations. Some letters cite the evaluations verbatim, others use abridged versions or just choice excerpts. Some deans' letters include histograms depicting the grade distributions in courses and rotations, and marking the student's position on each histogram.

► **Special activities.** Here the dean has an opportunity to highlight your extracurricular activities and any outstanding achievements. These passages often read like portraiture or—at worst—caricature.

► **Summary paragraph.** This section is usually read first by the residency selection committee. It is typically a concise synopsis of the Dean's letter, and likewise often provides a comparative analysis of your performance, whether through a class rank, class percentile or buzzwords that function to cluster or single out students (Table 5–4).

**KNOW WHAT INFLUENCE YOU HAVE OVER YOUR DEAN'S LETTER.**

The letter can be written without your input. At the other extreme, your school might ask you to proofread the letter for typos and factual errors, or even allow you limited editorial privileges with regard to the content. Other schools will consider it a federal offense if you so much as sneak a peek at your dean's letter. If the dean's office calls you in for a talk with the dean, be sure to bring along your CV or personal statement. In any event, ask savvy seniors and your student affairs office about the structure of the typical dean's letter from your institution, and what role you can expect to play in its final form. Table 5–5 presents a tongue-in-cheek view of the code words found in the dean's letter.

If you have the opportunity to review your dean's letter, check it carefully for accuracy, grammar, and spelling, and for the presence of all your clerkship evaluations (no need to point out any weak ones that might be missing). If you have not already done so, do not hesitate to visit your dean of students to discuss any evaluations that you believe to be unfair, inaccurate or even malicious. If your school gives you the opportunity to edit the content of your dean's letter, **grab it!** Medical schools want their graduates to do well, and few can market you like you yourself. Make sure the dean's letter emphasizes your strong points in detail, while tactfully expressing con-

| | **TABLE 5-4. Examples of buzz words used in deans' letters.** | | |
|---|---|---|---|
| **Best** | Recommend in highest terms | Outstanding | Strongest of year |
| ↓ | Recommend very highly | Excellent | Very strong |
| | Recommend highly | Very good | Strong |
| **Worst** | Recommend | Good | Good |

**TABLE 5-5. The unofficial guide to translating the Dean's letter[1]**

| What the Dean Says | What the Dean Really Means |
|---|---|
| Sensitive | Cries easily |
| Very sensitive | Cries on rounds |
| Very cooperative | Easy; will work extra nights |
| Relatively good | Wouldn't want him/her for my doctor |
| Sensitive to patients' needs | Steals food from their trays |
| Extremely capable | A little better than average |
| Well-liked | His/her mom always spoke well of him/her |
| Extremely conscientious | Probably paranoid |
| Assertive | A real SOB |
| Self-motivated | Obnoxious |
| Outstanding integrity | On parole; is watching every step |
| Enthusiastic | Hebephrenic |
| Grasps new concepts quickly | Basically stupid, but flexible |
| Highly satisfactory | Extremely average |
| Compulsive, goal-oriented | Obnoxious, but no more than average |
| Recommend with confidence | Glad to get him/her out of our school |
| Recommend with reservation | Glad to get him/her out of our school |
| Look forward to watching this individual mature in his/her career | Sure hope the fool improves |
| Will be an asset to your program | Don't call us, we'll call you! |

[1] Adapted, with permission, from the *New England Journal of Medicine*.

cerns about negative material that may have made its way into the collection. Everyone has suffered a premature or harsh judgment made by someone who doesn't really know them. If you have one or two isolated "pans" in your record, a sympathetic dean may be willing to soften or delete them.

Most deans' letters are mailed out on the first of November, a date agreed upon by the council of deans. A few send out their information earlier. For this reason, it's a good idea to confirm your dean's mailing date. Then, provide your dean's office with your list of programs with addresses (as well as stamps and envelopes if necessary) **well before the mailing date.** Check with the office a day after the mailing date to confirm that your letters have indeed been sent.

## LETTERS OF RECOMMENDATION

Along with your deans' letter, your letters of recommendation are vital to the success of your application. Take the time to select your letter writers wisely, and provide them with the materials they may need to refresh their memories when they write their recommendations.

### When Should I Start Requesting Letters of Recommendation?

You can ask for letters after completing any significant clinical or research experience. Most students start collecting letters during the third year of medical school. If you did well on a third-year clerkship, ask the attending to write a letter and put it aside while you are still fresh in his or her mind, keeping in mind that the letter can be modified later to reflect your specialty choice and career goals. In general, whenever you ask for a letter, give the writer at least four weeks to write the letter and mail it off.

## How Do I Get a Strong Letter of Recommendation?

When you solicit letters of recommendation, there are a few steps you can take to maximize your chances of getting the strongest possible letters. First, go to the clerkship office and read the evaluations that your potential reference wrote about you during your rotation. The strength and eloquence of the writer's evaluation will certainly be reflected in any later letter written on your behalf.

Second, when asking for a letter of recommendation, phrase your request carefully. This precaution may reduce your vulnerability to weak letters. Tact and discretion are all the more important late in the game when clerkship evaluations may not be available to you. You can, for example, ask the person, "Do you think you know me well enough to write me a **strong** letter of recommendation?" If the potential referee does not feel comfortable writing you a strong letter, he or she can take the graceful exit you provided, saying, "Actually, I don't believe I know you well enough. Perhaps you should ask someone else." Then you are free to request a letter from another attending or faculty member who may provide you with a better reference.

Third, meet in person with the writer **before** he or she sits down to compose the letter, in order to discuss your choice of specialty and your career goals. Provide your letter writer with a copy of your personal statement, your CV, the names and addresses of the programs to which you are applying, (or a computer diskette, if the writer wants to do a mail merge), a set of stamps, and possibly a copy of their earlier evaluation of you if the comments were impressive and you would not mind having them recycled in the letter.

Some attendings will draft a letter of recommendation and offer you the chance to read it and either decline or accept it. If the letter is not as strong as you had hoped, you may decline it as long as you have better letters coming (Table 5–6). If the attending does not offer to show it to you, you may tactfully try the direct approach and ask if they would mind if you saw the letter or be less direct and ask to have a copy for your files. Many writers view this as

PREPPING FOR RECOMMENDATION: ALWAYS MEET WITH YOUR WRITERS IN PERSON TO DISCUSS THEIR LETTERS.

| TABLE 5-6. Signs of a strong or weak letter. | |
|---|---|
| **Strong** | **Weak** |
| Typewritten on official letterhead and personally signed | Handwritten on plain paper and photocopied |
| Handwritten postscript with political schmoozing a big plus | Signed by an assistant or signature photocopied |
| Lengthy | Short |
| Detailed description of fund of knowledge, clinical skill, and past performance | Vague. Focuses on marginally relevant personality traits or work habits (eg,"He was punctual and well dressed.") |
| Frequent personal references | Lack of familiarity |
| Unconditional praise | Lukewarm praise; qualifications of any kind (but, except, etc.) |

a reasonable request since letters of recommendation often get lost and you may end up faxing a copy of the missing letter to the program to complete your file. If you are applying in a competitive specialty or you are a marginal candidate, then you may want copies of your letters of recommendation handy for the Scramble in case you do not match. Others still maintain that their letters should be strictly confidential. If you see the letter early and the letter is unfavorable (Table 5–6), you may decide to withhold program addresses. However, make sure you have someone else to go to for a letter. Even if letters have been sent, you should be aware of the content of the letters just in case it pops up during the residency interview.

ASK LETTER WRITERS TO SEND A COPY TO THE DEAN'S OFFICE TO HAVE READY IN CASE YOU MUST ENTER THE SCRAMBLE.

*REC: Family medicine? ER? Peds?*

## Whom Should I Ask for Letters of Recommendation?

You should look for the following characteristics in all your letter writers if possible. He or she should be someone who:

► Will write you a strong letter

► Knows you well in a clinical setting

► Is well-established in the field (in order of desirability: chairman, professor, clinical instructor)

► Works in your specialty choice or in a related field

► Trained at or is well-known at your top-choice program

If given the choice of a letter from a well-connected figure who does **not** know you well, or from a lesser-known attending who is familiar with you and your work, give priority to the person who knows you better. Unfortunately, many students request letters from less than optimal sources (Table 5–7). Letters from research mentors are acceptable if you already have two clinical letters and you have a strong interest in doing research in the future. Make sure it's from someone with whom you have done considerable work (ie, more than one summer). Letter selection also depends on the type of program you are applying to. It borders on excessive, but some applicants actually pick and choose from among five or more letter writers, depending upon the characteristics of each program on their list.

**TABLE 5-7. Sub-optimal sources for letters of recommendation.**

| |
| --- |
| Residents |
| Preclinical professors |
| Family, friends |
| Community figures |
| Previous employers |

## TRANSCRIPTS

Before you have your transcripts (medical school, and in some cases, undergraduate) mailed out, request some student copies to review for errors and completeness. Try to get your transcript requests to the registrar's office a few weeks before you send out your applications (September for most NRMP applicants). If you should receive additional excellent grades after the transcripts are mailed, send out updated transcripts.

DON'T FORGET TO PROOFREAD YOUR TRANSCRIPT.

## PHOTO

Most applications reserve a space for a passport size photograph. Others will ask you to bring a photo when you interview. Though it is illegal to require a photograph with the application, it is better to comply unless you bear a striking resemblance to Darth Vader. Consider going to a studio for professional photography, and have color prints developed unless specified otherwise. If the pictures turn out well, you can send a 5x7 copy to your parents or your significant other.

## APPLICATION STATUS

Early match applicants will receive a letter from CAS detailing the documents it has received and the programs that the application has been sent to. ERAS applicants can track the status of their applications through the Applicant Document Tracking System (ADTS). The ADTS will show you a list of your selected programs, along with the dates that the documents were uploaded by the dean's office and downloaded by the residency program.

Non-ERAS residency programs have a variety of methods for acknowledging receipt of your application material, ranging from no response to a letter acknowledging receipt of the application form that checks any missing materials. Overall, it's up to you to track your application materials. This can easily be done by including a stamped, self-addressed postcard that notes receipt of your application and has a checklist for missing material (Figure 5–5). For the acknowledgment postcard to do its job, make sure that arrangements for all other materials are made well before sending in your applications. The exception is the dean's letter, which is usually mailed out November 1.

**Alternative Methods of Application Tracking.** Unfortunately, the enclosed postcard only works if the overworked program secretary is in a mood to mail it back. Return receipt service available from the post office or express mail with tracking numbers are better but more expensive ways of tracking your applications. If you prefer, wait a few weeks after your application has been sent in, then call the program to check on your file (especially if you did not receive an application completed postcard). Not only will the contact person at the program verify if your file is complete, he or she may have advance word on your interview status. Most programs don't mind a phone call, as long as your manner is courteous and professional. Remember: the impression you make on the office staff may tip the balance toward or against your application.

APPLICATION "RECEIVED"
DOES NOT EQUAL
APPLICATION "COMPLETE."
CONFIRM BY MAIL
OR PHONE THAT ALL
APPLICATIONS ARE
COMPLETE WELL IN ADVANCE
OF INTERVIEWS.

### FIGURE 5-5

This is to acknowledge receipt of your application.
___ Your application is **complete.**
___ Your application is **not** complete. We are missing the following item(s):

___ Dean's letter
___ Transcript
___ Letter from Dr. Alpha
___ Letter from Dr. Beta
___ Letter from Dr. Gamma
___ Other _____

_____ _____
*(You fill in the blank)*
Program                                    Date

Sample application status postcard.

# REFERENCES

AAMC-ERAS website (http://www.aamc.org/~eras).

Greenburg A et al: Letters of recommendation for surgical residencies: What they say and what they mean. *J Surg Res* 1994;56:192.

Hunt DD et al: Characteristics of dean's letters in 1981 and 1992. *Acad Med* 1993;68;905.

Leiden LI, Miller GD: National survey of writers of dean's letters for residency applications. *J Med Educ* 1986;61:943.

Medschool.com website (http://www.medschool.com).

San Francisco Residency Match website (http://www.sfmatch.org).

*Vanderbilt School of Medicine Guide to Residency Applications.* Vanderbilt University, 1994.

Wagoner NE et al: Factors used by program directors to select residents. *J Med Educ* 1986;61:12.

Wagoner NE, Suriano, JR: Program directors' responses to a survey on variables used to select residents in a time of change. *Acad Med* 1999;74:51.

Zagumny MJ, Rudolph J: Comparing medical students' and residency directors' ratings of criteria used to select residents. *Acad Med* 1992;67:613.

REC Family medicine?
ER?
Peds?
— u honors
— nis award
— Pass Peds

# The Curriculum Vitae

In the world of applications and interviews, the CV or the resumé is the equivalent of the 1-minute bullet patient presentation. It should be concise yet complete. A well-written CV places a succinct, factual yet positive account of your academic, career, and extracurricular accomplishments at the fingertips of the residency director. The CV works with the rest of your application to win you an interview. After that, the rest is up to you. You should create a preliminary CV early in the process (ie, during May through July) so that your letter writers can use it as a reference source. You will also want it close at hand as you work on your personal statement. You can fine-tune and expand your CV at the end of the summer.

ERAS requires applicants to enter CV information directly into the program, without the option to make changes to style and formal items such as fonts, styles, and margins. However, you should still create a professionally formatted CV for several reasons. First, most letter writers will require a CV that they can use as a reference source. Also, when attending interviews, many interviewers will request to see a copy of your CV. So even though you cannot include your personally designed CV as a part of your initial application, you should still spend the time needed to create an organized, professional and attractive CV. Students applying to specialties with match processes outside the NRMP, such as neurology, neurosurgery, ophthalmology, otolaryngology, and urology will use their CV as a part of their application since they will not be applying through the ERAS program.

## WHAT'S IN A CV?

A CV typically can include the following elements:

- **Name and address:** Stick with the same name that you use in your applications, dean's letter, transcripts, and correspondence with the programs and the matching service. Make sure you include an address, a phone number, and an e-mail address through which program directors can reach you during the entire interview season. Give a secondary address and phone number (ie, parents') if no one is at your primary address when you are away during the interviewing season.

- **Objective:** A terse, 1-sentence statement of your residency and career goals. Include only if your career goals are not readily apparent to the residency director (eg, a fellowship and academic practice in hand surgery after a residency in orthopedic surgery).

▶ **Education:** List all major or medically related educational experiences from the present through college. Dual graduate degrees (eg, MD/PhD, MD/MPH, MD/JD) are particularly impressive and should be highlighted. Include the name and place of the institution, your area of study, dates of enrollment, type of degree received, and honors bestowed at graduation (eg, graduating cum laude). If you are a U.S. senior medical student, list your expected graduation date.

▶ **Honors:** Include any awards and scholarships that you have received during your med school years, as well as the most important awards and scholarships from your undergraduate years. If you did well in school or on the boards, list your honors and board scores.

▶ **Publications:** Catalog any abstracts and papers published or submitted for publication. Format each publication as a detailed bibliographic reference. Also list research presented or talks given at conferences/poster sessions.

▶ **Extracurricular activities:** Include the most important long-term activities you were involved in during medical school or recently, if you have already graduated. This category would include such things as community service projects, committee work, participation in student organizations, etc.

▶ **Work experience:** List all major or medically related work experiences, whether paid or volunteer (eg, paramedic work, nursing). Include dates of work experience.

▶ **Personal:** List hobbies and interests that define you. Also mention any special qualifications or skills that might enhance your effectiveness as a house officer (eg, foreign language training, knowledge of sign language for the deaf, computer skills, etc.).

The phrase "references available upon request" seen in most non-medical CVs is redundant, since letters of recommendation are a required element of the application. Sometimes it helps to list your references by name in the CV, especially if they are particularly illustrious and widely respected.

Note that certain information is **not** appropriate for a medical professional CV (Table 6–1). You may have to consider including information about citizenship or visa status if you are an IMG.

## HOW DO I PUT TOGETHER MY CV?

Study the sample CVs starting on page 109 to get a feel for the appearance you want in your finished CV. On a word processor, fill in information under the categories listed above. If you have nothing to say under a category, do not include it. Note that most CVs will start with "Name/Address" and "Education" and end with "Personal." In the middle, however, you can rearrange the order of the remaining categories to emphasize strengths and downplay less impressive areas. Refer to the sample CVs to see various designs available.

After inputting the basic information, edit your document into a professional and attractive format and style using the sample CVs as a guide. See Table 6–2 for specific writing tips. Make sure that your CV is pleasing to the eye (Table 6–3). Keep your language terse; sentence fragments often suf-

---

*Handwritten margin notes:*
- JHU honors
- Tennis award
- High Pass: Peds
- Boards

---

**TABLE 6-1. Information not appropriate in a CV.**

Birth place and date

Citizenship status (except IMG)

Marital status

Names of spouse and family members

High school education/accomplishments *(no volunteer)*

---

**ARRANGE THE ELEMENTS OF YOUR CV TO HIGHLIGHT YOUR STRONG POINTS.**

| **TABLE 6-2. CV writing tips.** |
| --- |
| • Organize categories to highlight strengths. |
| • If you're an older applicant, try to avoid unexplained gaps in timeline. |
| • Use terse, precise, and vivid language. |
| • Create parallel structure in lists (eg, each item in a list starts with a verb). |
| • Follow consistent punctuation rules. |
| • Follow consistent capitalization rules. |
| • When in doubt, consult a style manual or a professional editor. |

fice. Use vivid nouns and active verbs (Tables 6–4, 6–5) to demonstrate strength, enthusiasm, and initiative. Pay **very** careful attention to style and punctuation. While no one expects medical students to take graduate seminars in English grammar and syntax, blunders in these areas won't help your application. Medicine is a detail oriented specialty, and sloppiness can be interpreted as evidence of carelessness or lack of motivation. If you have any further doubts, refer to the sample CVs, show your draft to a friend with good writing skills, or consult a manual of style such as Strunk and White's *Elements of Style.*

Ask your career adviser and at least one other person to read the CV and provide feedback on the following: appearance/legibility, ease of reading, grammar, punctuation, and style (Table 6–3). After making any necessary revisions, make copies from a laser printer onto high-quality paper. Choose a heavy cotton bond paper in white or a neutral color to make your CV stand out in a pile (Table 6–6). Alternatively, you can make a master copy and take it to a copy center, choose your paper (most of these places have a good selection of appropriate colors and bond weights), and make high-quality photocopies on the spot.

If you don't have access to a computer or laser printer, don't know how to use one, or just freeze when it comes to putting your life history on paper, you can always have your CV created and reproduced by a copy center (eg, Kinko's) or by a resume specialist as listed in the Yellow Pages. It's true that an overworked secretary in the student affairs office may assist you or do the job for free, but professional service is usually more effective and efficient.

**AVOID THE COLORS OF A RAINBOW.**

| **TABLE 6-3. CV layout and design tips.** |
| --- |
| • Allow for generous margins (1–1.5 inches). |
| • Limit resumé to 2 pages. |
| • Avoid splitting a section when going from page 1 to page 2. |
| • Try a serif font as the base text font for better legibility. Save sans serif for section headers. |
| • Do not go below 12 points for font size and 14 points for leading. |
| • Stay true to your fonts. Too many is distracting and gaudy. |
| • Be consistent with section headers in style and formatting. |
| • Boldface your name in any publications cited. |
| • Use boldface, small caps, italics, and bullet symbols sparingly. Avoid underlining. |
| • Print CV on a laser printer. |
| • Print CV on a heavyweight, cotton bond paper. Use a neutral color (eg, ivory). |
| • Make sure the finished CV photocopies well. |

| TABLE 6-4. Action verbs. | | | |
|---|---|---|---|
| accelerated | directed | lectured | reorganized |
| accomplished | effected | led | revamped |
| achieved | elucidated | maintained | reviewed |
| adapted | established | managed | revised |
| administered | evaluated | mastered | scheduled |
| analyzed | examined | motivated | set up |
| approved | expanded | operated | solved |
| attained | expedited | organized | streamlined |
| clarified | facilitated | originated | structured |
| completed | found | participated | studied |
| conceived | generated | performed | supervised |
| conducted | improved | pinpointed | supported |
| controlled | increased | planned | synthesized |
| coordinated | influenced | proposed | taught |
| created | implemented | proved | trained |
| delegated | initiated | provided | translated |
| demonstrated | instructed | recommended | used |
| designed | interpreted | reduced | won |
| developed | launched | reinforced | wrote |

## KISSES OF DEATH

Lastly, we are providing you with a handy checklist of no-nos for CVs. Any one of these can be a killer. To repeat advice given earlier, have your adviser and another competent person read your CV, with particular attention to the following:

- **Unprofessional appearance.** Do **not** write your CV by hand or use a typewriter. Dot matrix is also dead. Laser printing at 300 dpi is now the standard; 600 dpi laser output, also readily available, is slightly better. If you find a mistake on the CV, no matter how minor, print out a new, corrected version. Do **not** make corrections, handwritten or typed, on the CV. Use only high-quality, heavyweight bond paper.

- **Inaccuracies or exaggerations.** Present your talents and accomplishments in the best light possible, but do not misrepresent them. Residency directors have many ways of verifying your claims. Even a minor "misrepresentation" can have a major impact on your credibility.

- **Too lengthy.** Do not exceed two pages in length unless you have really stellar experience and an impressive list of publications to justify more space. Remember that this is a capsule summary of your career to date, not an extended autobiography.

- **Misspellings, poor grammar.** These unspectacular mistakes will only contribute to an image of carelessness or incompetence, particularly since most word processors make it easy to check spelling and grammar.

- **Weak writing.** Verbosity kills; keep your sentences short and succinct. Specifics count; the more precisely you can describe your experience, the better the reader can picture—and appreciate—what you say. Stay away from bland nouns and passive verbs.

| TABLE 6-6. Appropriate colors and patterns for CV paper. |
|---|
| White |
| Ivory |
| Beige |
| Light gray |
| Flannel pattern |
| Speckle pattern |

| TABLE 6-5. Concrete nouns and positive modifiers. | | | |
|---|---|---|---|
| ability | competent | proficient | technical |
| actively | consistent | qualified | unique |
| capacity | effectively | resourceful | versatile |
| competence | pertinent | substantially | vigorous |

**FIGURE 6–1A**

This applicant has a well-rounded CV with no real outstanding achievements. But because he is applying to several academic training programs, he chooses to list his research experience first.

---

**WILLIAM BRADFORD THOMAS**
325 Drummond Lane
Louisville, KY 40322
(512) 555-7457

---

### EDUCATION

| 1991-Present | **University of Louisville School of Medicine.** M.D. anticipated May 1995. |
| 1987-1991 | **Centre College of Kentucky.** B.S., Biology and Psychology, *magna cum laude*. |

### RESEARCH

| Summer, 1992 | **Summer Research Fellow.** Stefan Maguire, PhD, Hormone Research Institute. Elucidated the role of glutamic acid decarboxylase in the autoimmune pathogenesis of insulin dependent diabetes mellitus. |
| Summer, 1990 | **Research Assistant.** Richard Woodbridge, MD, University of Kentucky Medical Research Building. Analyzed flow characteristics of IV infusion pumps to evaluate their accuracy in removing outflow of spent dialysate and ultrafiltrate. |

> *Do not forget to list your principal investigator*

### PUBLICATIONS

**W. Thomas** and S. Maguire. "Is $GAD_{65}$ localized to synaptic-like vesicles in ß-pancreatic cells?" 1992 School of Medicine Research Poster Session.

R. Woodbridge, **W. Thomas,** D. Arnold, J. Funk. "Accuracy of IV Pumps in CAVHD." *American Society for Artificial Internal Organs: 1991 Abstracts,* 1991, p. 78.

> *Text is indented to keep clean, vertical look*

### HONORS & AWARDS

| 1991 | **Michael Ryan Biology Prize.** Centre College. |
| 1991 | **Jeffrey Scott McBride Leadership Award.** Centre College. |
| 1990 | **Phi Beta Kappa** |
| 1987-1991 | **Trustee Scholarship.** Half tuition merit scholarship. |

---

Sample CV No. 1

*Honors:*
*Graduated c̄ honors at JHU*

**FIGURE 6-1B**

WILLIAM BRADFORD THOMAS

*EXTRACURRICULAR*

1994-Present   **Faculty Student Network Committee.** Organized events and meetings for faculty advisers and medical students.

**School of Medicine Representative, Registration Fee Committee.** Committee allocates student fees to student organizations and services.

1992-1993   **Peer Counselor, Campus Health.** Provided counseling and support for first-year medical students.

1991-Present   **Homeless Health Clinic.** Evaluated and treated homeless patients as medical volunteer in homeless shelter.

1991-1992   **Vice-president, AMA–Medical Student Section Chapter.** Organized health fairs and guest speakers for medical school chapter.

*PROFESSIONAL MEMBERSHIPS*

1991-Present   **American Medical Association, Medical Student Section**

1994-Present   **American Academy of Pediatrics, Medical Student Section**

*PERSONAL*

Proficient in American sign language.
Hobbies include volleyball, jogging. *tennis, teaching, running*

> Use "action" verbs to give an active tone

---

*Extracurricular*

2001, 2002 (April):    MS Walk at Nottingham High School

2003    Health fair at ~~midd~~ Bellevue elementary school. Promoted Healthy Eating.

2003, July    Walk for Life (cancer) at Ithaca High School. Relay for Life. American Cancer Society.

Look at resumé for more

**FIGURE 6-2A**

This CV emphasizes the applicant's considerable research accomplishments. If she were applying to mostly clinical programs, she might alternatively choose to highlight her strong extracurricular activities.

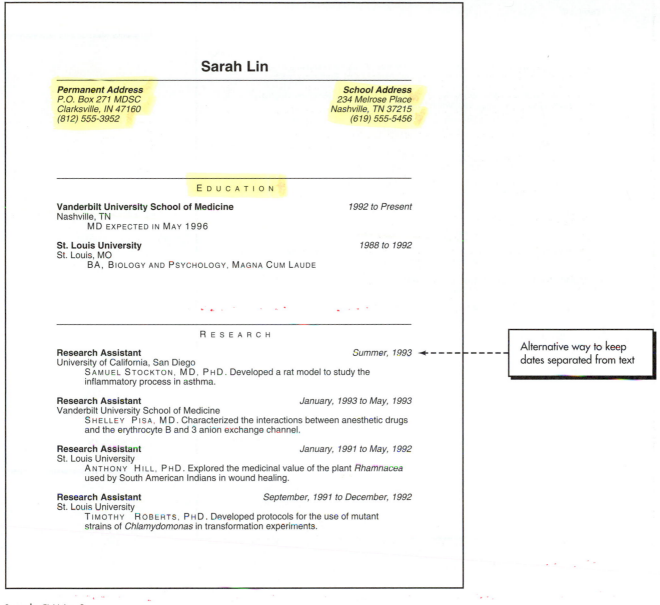

# Sarah Lin

| **Permanent Address** | **School Address** |
|---|---|
| P.O. Box 271 MDSC | 234 Melrose Place |
| Clarksville, IN 47160 | Nashville, TN 37215 |
| (812) 555-3952 | (619) 555-5456 |

### EDUCATION

**Vanderbilt University School of Medicine**      *1992 to Present*
Nashville, TN
  MD EXPECTED IN MAY 1996

**St. Louis University**      *1988 to 1992*
St. Louis, MO
  BA, BIOLOGY AND PSYCHOLOGY, MAGNA CUM LAUDE

### RESEARCH

**Research Assistant**      *Summer, 1993*
University of California, San Diego
  SAMUEL STOCKTON, MD, PHD. Developed a rat model to study the inflammatory process in asthma.

**Research Assistant**      *January, 1993 to May, 1993*
Vanderbilt University School of Medicine
  SHELLEY PISA, MD. Characterized the interactions between anesthetic drugs and the erythrocyte B and 3 anion exchange channel.

**Research Assistant**      *January, 1991 to May, 1992*
St. Louis University
  ANTHONY HILL, PHD. Explored the medicinal value of the plant *Rhamnacea* used by South American Indians in wound healing.

**Research Assistant**      *September, 1991 to December, 1992*
St. Louis University
  TIMOTHY ROBERTS, PHD. Developed protocols for the use of mutant strains of *Chlamydomonas* in transformation experiments.

Alternative way to keep dates separated from text

Sample CV No. 2

**FIGURE 6-2B**

*Sarah Lin*                                                                                          2    ◄ - - - - - -

Include a header if your CV has 2 pages

P U B L I C A T I O N S

C. Anand, V. Beck, T. Carusi, **S. Lin,** contributing author. *Solutions Guide and Study Manual to Retired and Self-Test Questions,* Ashland, OH: Butterfield, 1995.

**S. Lin,** A. Hill. "Wound healing properties of the *Rhamnacea* plant." *American Journal of Herbal Medicine,* June 1993, Vol. 22, No. 6, pp. 210-212.

E X T R A C U R R I C U L A R

**St. Thomas Catholic Charity Services**                                   *1994 to Present*
Taught English to Vietnamese refugees and served as interpreter for social workers.

**A Room in the Inn**                                                                     *1993 to Present*
Prepared and served meals in a homeless soup kitchen.

**Morari School Project**                                                               *1992 to 1993*
Organized health science presentations for elementary school children.

**Asian American Medical Student Association**                        *1992 to Present*
Promoted community and school awareness of health care and Asian culture.

**St. Louis University Student Admissions Committee**              *1990 to 1992*
Recruited prospective students and aided in the selection process.

**Cultural Celebration Committee**                                           *1989 to 1992*
Helped organize an annual undergraduate cultural fair.

P E R S O N A L

Fluent in Cantonese.
Hobbies include ethnic cuisine and gardening.   ◄ - - - - - - - - - - - - - - -

Be ready to discuss anything on your CV in detail

**FIGURE 6-3A**

This applicant has an impressive number of awards and honors. Because she is entering family practice, she emphasizes her community service experience and lists her research on the second page.

## Jacquelyn H. Lemmon

**School Address**
576 London Road, Apt. #5
Tucson, AZ 85719
(602) 555-7456

**Permanent Address**
2145 Red Valley Drive
Danville, TN 34205
(615) 555-5760

*Education*

| | |
|---|---|
| 1992–1996 | UNIVERSITY OF ARIZONA SCHOOL OF MEDICINE<br>M.D. expected in May, 1996 |
| 1988–1992 | WASHINGTON UNIVERSITY<br>B.S. in Engineering & Policy |

*Honors & Awards*

| | |
|---|---|
| 1994 | BRISTOL-MYERS SQUIBB SCHOLAR |
| 1993–1996 | MICROBES AND DEFENSE SOCIETY |
| 1993 | DIABETES SUMMER RESEARCH GRANT<br>Awarded by Diabetes Research and Training Center. |
| 1993 | SUMMER RESEARCH GRANT<br>Awarded by American Society for Lasers in Medicine and Surgery. |
| 1992–1996 | JUSTIN POTTER SCHOLARSHIP<br>Merit award based on leadership potential. |
| 1991–1992 | MORTAR BOARD HONOR SOCIETY |
| 1988–1992 | JOHN B. ERVIN SCHOLARSHIP |

*Extracurricular*

| | |
|---|---|
| 1992–Present | STUDENT NATIONAL MEDICAL ASSOCIATION<br>Promoted health care and minority issues. Served as co-chairperson and treasurer of Arizona chapter. |
| 1994–Present | TUCSON CARES<br>Made lecture presentations on HIV/AIDS to the general public on behalf of agency, which serves HIV/AIDS population. |

All-caps is an alternative to boldfaced text.

Sample CV No. 3.

**FIGURE 6–3B**

*Jacquelyn H. Lemmon*

**Extracurricular,** *continued*

1992–Present      VARIOUS SERVICE ACTIVITIES
Participated in several community service activities including Inn for
the Homeless, Habitat for Humanity, wheelchair ramp construction,
role model activities for black youth.

1992      SUBSTANCE ABUSE AND PREVENTION PROGRAM
Counseled high-risk youth as part of a first-year elective.

**Research**

March–August, 1995      RESEARCH ELECTIVE, CENTERS FOR DISEASE CONTROL
AND PREVENTION
Preceptor Richard Woodbridge, MD. Designed methods for
collecting and organizing for international importations data.
Collected and analyzed 1995 data with comparison to data collected
from 1986 to 1994.

1994      RESEARCH ASSISTANT
Preceptor George Sherman, MD. Characterized lymphocytic
migration in RSV-infected mice. Results presented at National
Medical Fellowships Research Seminar in February, 1995.

Summer, 1993      SUMMER RESEARCH FELLOW
Preceptor Lou Ritter, MD. Tested various pulse structures of the
electron laser to evaluate its efficacy in bone ablation.

Summer, 1993      RESEARCH ASSISTANT
Preceptor Lou Ritter, MD. Developed optimal laser firing patterns to
achieve minimal thermal buildup in a collagen-based target. Results
presented to the Arizona Diabetes Research Training Center.

**Personal**

Hobbies include jogging, piano, swimming.

2

> A good way to present multiple small activities.

**FIGURE 6-4**

Both a 1-page CV and a 2-page CV are acceptable. Because everything is on 1 page, the order of categories is not as important.

Thicker line adds style

### Stephanie L. Locke
2733 Forrest Avenue
Knoxville, TN 37225
(502) 555-5555

*Education*
1992 –
Present

**University of Tennessee School of Medicine**     Knoxville, TN
M.D. anticipated in May, 1996

List location of school if not obvious

**Indiana University**                                  Indianapolis,
B.S. with Honors, *magna cum laude*
Molecular Genetics with minor in Chemistry

*Honor*
1992 – 1996

**Francis Pederson Scholarship.** Full-tuition, merit and need-based award.

Explain honors and awards as needed

1994

**Amos Christie Pediatric Summer Fellowship**

1993 –
Present

**Microbes and Defense Society.** Honor society for excellence in microbiology and immunology.

**Phi Beta Kappa**

*Activities*
1994 – 1996

**Committee on Women's Issues.** Co-Chairperson for Volunteer Activities. Promoted public awareness of women's issues in medicine.

1993 –
Present

**Decisions Pathway Program.** Assisted women in a Tennessee prison through substance abuse rehabilitation.

1993 –

**Center for Health Services Board.** Nominating Committee Member, 1994-1995; Project Advisory Committee Member, 1993-1994.

**American Medical Student Association.**

*Employment*
Summer
1994

**Clinical Clerk, Amos Christie Pediatric Summer Fellowship.** Evaluated patients in the pediatric acute care clinic, the newborn nursery, and the cardiology clinic.

Include major jobs and employment related to teaching and health

1990 – 1992

**Academic Assistant & Tutor, Indiana University Minority Office.** Tutored students in inorganic chemistry. Organized tutoring program by matching students to appropriate tutors.

*Personal*

Conversational in Spanish.
Hobbies include aerobics, cooking, reading, and

Vertical line is an alternative to horizontal lines in other CVs

Sample CV No. 4.

# REFERENCES

"Resume Guidelines." Southworth Paper Company, 1995.
"Roadmap to the Match resource Center," Medschool.com website (http://www.medschool.com).

# The Personal Statement

**7**

Writing the personal statement can be excruciating. It's hard to start and harder yet to know exactly what the selection committee wants to read. A draft that feels inspired at the moment of composition often seems hokey 2 days later. As much as you might like to, you can't simply rehash your AMCAS personal statement, as it usually does not address the same issues covered by a good personal statement for the Match (ie, the traits of a good medical student are often different from those of a good house officer). In addition, despite all the trouble you take to write it, the personal statement is often seen by residency selection committees as an opportunity to weed out applicants. Thus, while an outstanding personal statement might salvage a mediocre application, a bad one can cripple a strong application.

Most selection committees tend to underanalyze (or ignore) personal statements during the high-volume screening process, and to over-scrutinize them during the knock-down, drag-out ranking sessions that follow the screening. It is common to see otherwise well-qualified applicants slide 20 to 40 positions on a rank list at the last minute because the selection committee suddenly perceived something in their personal statements as negative.

For this reason, do not take the personal statement lightly. It is the one part of the application over which you have **total** control, and your one chance for creative expression. Residency directors often use the personal statement to check for qualities not readily apparent from your application form—such as maturity, enthusiasm, thoughtfulness, humility, stability, and a willingness to learn. Note the characteristics that directors look for in future house officers; if your personal statement conveys these qualities, it will strengthen your application.

A GREAT PERSONAL STATEMENT MIGHT HELP AN APPLICATION, BUT A BAD ONE WILL KILL IT.

THE FOUR As OF A SUCCESSFUL HOUSE OFFICER: (1) ATTITUDE; (2) AFFABILITY; (3) AVAILABILITY; (4) ABILITY.

## GETTING STARTED

The keys to writing a good personal statement are to start early and to revise, revise, revise. You should finish the statement by September or October, so most people will write their personal statements over the summer between third and fourth years. The hardest part is just getting started. The easiest way to start is with brainstorming. Don't worry whether your ideas are original or even good; just write them down. There are certain elements that are covered in all personal statements. All are "revelation stories" to some degree—showing how your upbringing, life events, and intellectual interests have influenced your current specialty and career aspirations. Most residency directors want to understand an applicant's personal reasons for seeking to enter the specialty, as well as his or her professional goals.

We've taken the liberty of listing questions you should ask yourself when building your statement. Thoughtful answers to 2 or 3 of these questions should give you enough substance for a good first draft. The safest and most familiar topics include: (1) reasons for choosing a specialty; (2) career plans; (3) accomplishments; and (4) interests outside medicine. Note that each of these topics implies a different time frame and has its own tense (past, present, future, conditional, etc.). It is up to you to decide how much backtracking, present-day analysis, and future-gazing you would like to do.

**(1) What are my reasons for choosing the specialty?** Most committee members who will review your application are curious about your reasons for choosing their specialty. Most applicants discuss the nature of the work, the patient population, the intellectual challenges, or the desire to make a unique contribution to medicine. Mentioning financial and lifestyle reasons, though they may have played a part in your decision-making process, is a *faux pas* in a personal statement.

**(2) What are my career plans?** The overused party line is to talk in vague generalities about having a clinical practice with possibly some academic involvement. Be as specific as possible without antagonizing anyone who might be reading your statement. Think about discussing the fit between your career goals on the one hand and your disposition and personal goals on the other. An ability to articulate clear and realistic plans will give the reader the sense that you have a firm understanding of their specialty.

**(3) What accomplishments do I want to emphasize?** You can use part of your personal statement to highlight a noteworthy activity or achievement that might have otherwise escaped the notice of the selection committee. You can skim through your CV and dean's letter to pinpoint such achievements. Use them to demonstrate your desire to enter the specialty, reveal a positive personal quality, or illustrate your worthiness to enter the field. Avoid, however, the temptation to rehash your CV in your personal statement.

**(4) What outside interests do I have?** Selection committees need to be assured that, apart from working 100+-hour weeks during the tougher rotations, depriving yourself of sleep and exercise on a regular basis, and actually paying a medical school to do this, you are otherwise a semi-normal person. Touch on extracurricular interests to add depth to the presentation of your character, or to illustrate personal qualities (eg, participation in community activities indicates both a sense of responsibility and a capacity for active involvement).

**(5) What contributions can I make to the specialty and the residency program?** Hold forth about your love of teaching, years of leadership training, computer expertise, and rich parents eager to donate big bucks to the program (just kidding). As discussed above, these considerations can be brought out in the context of accomplishments, reasons for entering the specialty, or outside interests.

STAY AWAY FROM FINANCIAL AND LIFESTYLE REASONS IN A PERSONAL STATEMENT.

DO NOT REHASH YOUR CV IN THE PERSONAL STATEMENT.

## DAMAGE CONTROL

In addition, you can carefully use a personal statement to address one or more of the following concerns:

1. **How can I compensate for serious problems or weaknesses in my application?** If you recognize that your record contains a real blot, you may preempt the selection committee's concern. Here is a chance to defend your record and demonstrate your ability to learn from poor performances and negative incidents. However, be careful not to (1) sound defensive, or (2) dwell on the negative. Discussion of negatives can easily backfire, especially by drawing attention to something that might have otherwise passed unnoticed. Find yourself a trusted adviser to discuss both general strategy and the wording of the statement itself.

2. **Are there any remaining issues (outstanding problems) that I would like to discuss during an interview?** If you believe that you cannot adequately address certain concerns in a personal statement, you may choose to indicate that you would be more than happy to discuss them during the interview. Again, review this option with your adviser.

## START WRITING

1. **Take a few of your ideas and work them into a rough draft.** Understand what your target programs want to see and what you have to offer in return. Then, choose 1 or 2 topics from the preceding list, in addition to reasons for entering the specialty and future career plans, to anchor your personal statement. The prototypical statement has 4 to 6 paragraphs.

   Don't worry about quality or length at this point—most likely your finished personal statement will look nothing like this first draft. Just get something—anything—down on paper. If it's easier, start with your conclusion or in the middle. Don't worry too much about being original. If you've honestly considered your reasons for entering your specialty, that's okay. Saying something the way you really feel it will help keep it from sounding trite.

2. **Come back a few days later.** Reconsider what you want to say, and rework your statement. Repeat this step until your statement is somewhat presentable.

3. **Ask friends/family members/advisors to read it.** You may want to start with a close friend or family member who is a good writer. Your statement likely needs a lot of reorganization at this point, and you want help from someone who will take plenty of time on it. Also, you are less likely to be self-conscious about showing this early, flawed draft to someone close than to an advisor. Be sure, however, to show it to your advisor or to someone else in medicine at some point for comments and suggestions.

## PERSONAL STATEMENT TIPS

1. **Be straightforward in your writing.** It's perfectly safe and actually desirable. As in your CV, stick with active verbs; avoid passive sentence structures. Writing manifests personality; you want to come across as energetic and ready for action.

2. **Vary your wording and sentence structure with the help of a thesaurus.** Most good word processors have an on-line thesaurus. Spell out non-standard abbreviations and explain local jargon; otherwise avoid them.

3. **Edit and proofread your work carefully.** Use the spell-checker in your word processor, then read the statement word for word for misspellings, since a word processor cannot spell-check in context. Grammar checkers give mixed results but usually do no harm. A professional editor can be cheap ($10 to $25 per hour) and preferable, if you can find a good one.

4. **Don't crowd your page with too much text.** Allow generous page margins (1 to 1.5 inches) and adequate spacing between each line (a minimum leading of 13 to 14 points, for you word processor geeks). Don't forget to indent paragraphs and add at least a half line between each paragraph.

5. **Choose an appropriate font.** Stick to serif fonts (eg, Times Roman, Garamond). Sans serif fonts (eg, Helvetica, Arial) are more difficult to read and photocopy poorly.

6. **Get a second opinion.** Have your statement read at least by your adviser and a second person with writing and editing skills.

7. **Revise—to a reasonable extent.**

8. **Don't get lost in the shuffle.** If your personal statement is separate from your application, then put your name and your NRMP identification number on top of the statement.

9. **Don't skimp on printing.** Print the final copies on a laser printer if you are not using ERAS. If the personal statement is separate from the application, print it on the same paper you used for your CV.

## KISSES OF DEATH FOR A PERSONAL STATEMENT

Since the personal statement is your big opportunity to impress committee members with a winning combination of skills and talents, it's tempting to indulge in ruffles and flourishes of one kind or another. Every year students strive for ways to jazz up their statements. Unfortunately, most of them end up falling into one of the following traps:

**Self-congratulatory statements:** If you happen to be God's gift to medicine, it is much better to let other people say that for you in your letters of recommendation and the dean's letter. Your personal statement should radiate confidence and a sense of self-worth without straying into arrogance.

**Self-centered statements:** Don't let the reader drown in a sea of "I's." Overuse of the first person singular can be interpreted either as a sign of self-centeredness or as a lack of writing skill.

**Emotional stories:** Heart-tugging stories about personal experiences with patients, personal illness, or an illness in the family that illustrate your motivations, your understanding of medicine, or your professional/personal qualities can have a spectacular effect. Unless you're Michael Crichton, however (who never finished a residency anyway), writing medical melodrama carries the risk of the reader's not "buying" your experience. This is especially true if you assign too much emotional value or influence to a specific experience (eg, inflated humanism). Will the average program director

A STATEMENT SHOULD RADIATE CONFIDENCE AND SELF-WORTH, NOT ARROGANCE.

really believe that one experience with a patient revolutionized your outlook on medicine, let alone your whole philosophy of life?

If you do include a personal account, describe it in rich detail and bring it to a satisfactory conclusion. Residency directors may be annoyed by influential life experiences that are described in a trite, superficial or incomplete manner.

**Overgeneralizations:** Unsupported claims that you are hardworking, efficient, curious, etc. may ring hollow without specific examples to back them up. Let your accomplishments, activities, and patient experiences attest to your professional and personal traits. Make sure your letter writers have a copy of your personal statement so they can corroborate your strengths.

**Use of tired analogies:** Avoid trite metaphors, such as comparing medical school to a box of chocolates. Other overworked cliches include "life is a road/path," "life is a journey," and "life is a book." If you think you have a genuinely creative idea, have several reviewers read your draft for honest feedback.

**Gimmicky writing:** Sometimes students try to impress readers with their creative writing skills. For example, one applicant wrote his statement in the form of an admit note. Attempts at literary originality may lead to speculation about the existence of significant psychopathology rather than to an appreciation of the writer's uniqueness. But all this doesn't mean you have to be boring. A conventional statement can still project enthusiasm, vitality, and wit. Committees are by nature conservative.

**Inconsistencies:** Your statement should agree with the rest of your application. If your transcripts show you to be an average student, don't write about yourself as the next Einstein. Your statement should also jibe with itself. If you want to be a rural family practitioner, what evidence can you present to demonstrate your interest in rural health care?

**Long statements:** Unless you're going into psychiatry, limit your personal statement to 1 page. Residency directors who read hundreds of essays view 2-page statements as divine retribution for their past sins. If you're afraid you won't be able to fit all your topics within the limit, ask your adviser or a friend to check your writing style for conciseness; it may be that critical editing is all you need.

**Digressions:** Every sentence you write should count; it should be clear in purpose and content. There is no need or room to repeat yourself if you made your point the first time.

**Illegible statements:** Personal statements that have a crammed appearance or are otherwise hard to read will only trigger migraines in your readers. Review the previous section on proofreading and printing for specific pointers about your statement's visual appearance.

**Misspellings, poor grammar:** Although this seems to be an obvious pitfall, people stumble into it more often than you would expect. Don't weaken an otherwise good statement with typos or mistakes in usage. Run your statement through the spelling checker if you have a word processor, and ask at least 2 people (including your adviser) to proofread and critique your essay.

SAVE THE BOWL OF CHERRIES.

LONG STATEMENTS GET PENALIZED — NOT FAIR, BUT THAT'S LIFE.

WRITE, REWRITE, EDIT AND PROOFREAD.

## SAMPLE EXCERPTS

We have included excerpts from actual personal statements as examples of do's and don'ts for certain issues. Names and locations have been changed to protect the writers' identities, but otherwise you're reading what the residency directors read. Most of the applicants behind these statements matched at top-flight institutions across the country. The comments that accompany our examples are derived from the observations of several residency directors, admissions committee members, and a professional editor. We hope that the critiques will help you acquire a "feel" for good form as well as good content. Keep in mind, however, that no two residency directors (even in the same specialty) read a personal statement with the same opinions and preferences.

### Strong or Engaging Openings

**Example #1.** This applicant in emergency medicine draws on rich family and cultural traditions and values. A residency director reading this introduction is not only making the acquaintance of an applicant, they are learning about the applicant's entire value system.

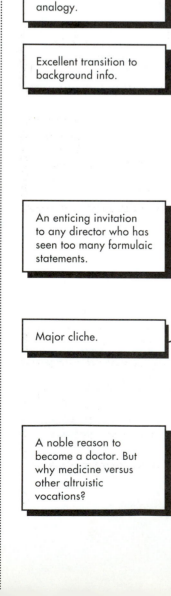

| Careful word choice enlivens an overused analogy.

| Excellent transition to background info.

> My great-grandfather once told me that everyone's life is like a book, full of chapters that are continually written and revised. Each life, each book, is unique, made so through the experiences and the actions of the person living. My personal anthology is no exception, having been enriched by the many people whom I have met. Through these experiences, I have strengthened my desire to enter a training program that will lead to a career in Emergency Medicine. Thus, begins a new chapter in my book. . . .

**Example #2.** A well done teaser for the rest of the statement. This family practice applicant weaves his sense of social responsibility and worldview (major family practice values) through a number of vivid experiences. Like a seductive movie trailer, the introduction pulls the reader in for more. The reader is left thinking, "This might be someone who would be fun to work with." The only way they will know for sure is by offering an interview.

| An enticing invitation to any director who has seen too many formulaic statements.

| Major cliche.

| A noble reason to become a doctor. But why medicine versus other altruistic vocations?

> I have always been interested in people's stories. This, and a deep-seated desire to help make the world a better place, have drawn me to the work I do. From working on a crew harvesting filberts to sitting down for a bowl of soup with a homeless friend, I have met many people, each one with a story, each story having something to teach me. Some of the wisest people I have met are very poor with little access to housing, education or health care. I get a lot out of listening to their stories; what do I give back? I first began to question the ethics of being a responsible listener when I went to Nicaragua as a Spanish interpreter. I was with a group of agronomists on a struggling agricultural cooperative nestled deep in the mountains of Matagalpa. The life was hard, but the work was fascinating and the setting beautiful. I finally got up the courage to ask the cooperative leader if I could stay longer. He smiled, "You gringos eat a lot. Now, maybe if you were a doctor. . . ." I chose to become a physician as a way to work intimately with people and hear their stories. But, just as importantly, it is a way to tangibly improve their lives.

**Example #3.** This applicant in anesthesiology successfully recycles a familiar travel theme with vivid imagery. The opening paragraph introduces a traveler enriched by his adventures. Unfortunately, we begin to sense that his actions have an unsettled, random quality.

While driving in the Mojave Desert, I turned off Highway 14 onto a dirt path. The road was crisscrossed by many other trails. Small hills blocked my view of what lay ahead on each road. Unable to see what each road led to, I randomly chose to drive along one road, then another, and then another. Every new direction possessed its own beauty and worth. One road revealed towering, sand-carved cliffs with striated bands of crimson, orange, and tan spotted with turquoise. Another road led to a lone Joshua tree standing majestically in the desert grass. Each new path inspired a new thought. I have had a similar experience in medicine.

> One hopes his choice of specialty was more deliberate. Rewrite to show some method to this madness.

> Vivid! You feel like you're there.

> Weak tie-in to medicine.

**Example #4.** This applicant in orthopedic surgery wants to return to the Midwest after training at an East Coast medical school. He combines the family legacy of an immigrant background with the rustic, traditional values of Middle America. However, by playing up the Midwest, he runs the risk of turning off East and West Coast directors in a highly competitive specialty in which applicants often have to apply coast-to-coast to match.

Growing up in the small farming community of Vernon in east-central Indiana, I have experienced a spectrum of attitudes unique to a rural population. Folks here are down to earth, with simple, relaxed lifestyles. It was here where I have lived almost all my life, moving from Birmingham, Alabama, my birthplace, at 9 months of age. It was here where my father set up his urology practice 30 years ago, having come from abroad with little more than a dream for a successful future. It was here, amidst the cornfields and cattle which I could see from my bedroom window, that I grew up with my older sister and younger brother under a strict, coherent value system of hard work, motivation, dedication, and perseverance.

> Back off a little on the rural imagery here. We get the point.

> Nice way of associating yourself with a set of values. Stating the same directly can come off as presumptuous.

## Reasons for Entering Specialty

**Example #1.** The following comes close to being a model illustration of good organization and presentation of motivations for pursuing a specialty. The applicant is obviously comfortable discussing the specialty, and appears sincere in his enthusiasm without being patronizing. The writing is sparse, but neither dry nor flat.

I grew up with surgery in my blood, but it was not until the middle of my third year of medical school that I discovered that I wanted to practice orthopedic surgery. It was at this time that I was first exposed to orthopedic surgery at Springfield Memorial Hospital. My love of being in the operating room, combined with the very precise mechanical and technical nature of orthopedic surgery, sparked my interest in the field. Perhaps the feature that fascinates me the most about orthopedics is that it is both a craft and a science. I enjoy the "hands-on" nature of orthopedic surgery, both in clinic and in the operating room. I am also attracted to the diversity of orthopedic cases and the vast amount of di-

> A bit cliche.

> Note the number of concrete reasons why orthopedics appeals to him.

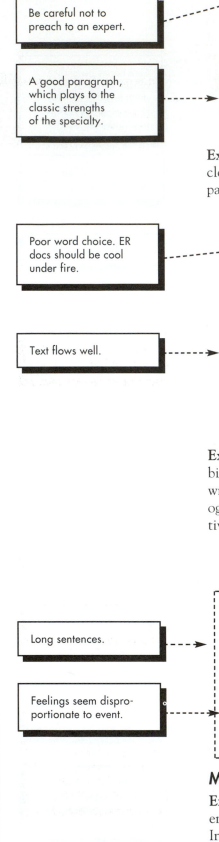

**Be careful not to preach to an expert.**

**A good paragraph, which plays to the classic strengths of the specialty.**

**Poor word choice. ER docs should be cool under fire.**

**Text flows well.**

**Long sentences.**

**Feelings seem disproportionate to event.**

rect patient contact. Treating patients of all age groups and both sexes, with a wide variety of problems encountered at work, in accidents, or during recreation, makes orthopedic surgery a very exciting specialty. Above all, although very demanding, I found my orthopedic surgery experiences to be the most rewarding and exhilarating in medical school. One can almost always do something specific and helpful for each patient, usually leading to a complete resolution of the patient's problem, so they can resume an active lifestyle.

**Example #2.** This is a tightly written paragraph in which the applicant clearly delineates her reasons for entering the specialty. The writing is fast-paced and precise, like the specialty she aspires to enter.

Although I have found all my clinical rotations interesting, I experienced the most excitement from my time in the emergency department. Emergency medicine offers me the opportunity to be at the forefront of medicine and to participate actively in making decisions right from the onset of patient care. The fast pace and the constant demand for rapid and clear thinking have always been attractive, as is the chance to be the first to see a patient, to gather all the relevant information, and then to ferret out the diagnosis. It is in the ED that I find a balanced mixture of the deliberative side of medicine with the more hands-on approach of surgery. But most of all, I enjoy relating to patients of different backgrounds, and eagerly look forward to the opportunity to care for the great variety of patients seen in emergency and acute settings.

**Example #3.** The following personal statement offers an interesting combination of professional and personal reasons for selecting the specialty. The writer risks conveying the impression, however, that he chose ophthalmology more as the result of a process of elimination than for its intrinsic attractiveness.

Although I have long been interested in ophthalmology, my choice of the specialty was not an easy one. Only after sampling what many other specialties had to offer did I realize that none suited me as well. The chance to combine extensive patient contact in a clinical setting with the need for surgical precision, attention to minute detail, and aptitude in the most advanced technology medicine has to offer is an obvious attraction of the specialty. Of all of my clinical experiences as a medical student at UCSF, however, none rivaled the pure emotion I felt during my senior clerkship in ophthalmology, as I watched the vision of a patient with a dense cataract I had examined in clinic be transformed from mere detection of hand motion to near normal the next day as a result of the ophthalmologist's expertise.

## Medicine as a Second Career

**Example #1.** In contrast to some second-career candidates, this applicant emphasizes the common ground between pediatrics and his previous career. In fact, the paragraph does not explain why he decided to make the career change.

For 5 years prior to medical school, I taught computer science in grades 2–12 at a private bilingual school. I loved working with children and their families and had the joy of seeing my students learn and grow over a number of years. These same preferences led me to an interest in pediatrics as a specialty. Pediatrics is a heady mixture of the exotic and the mundane, of glowing health and desperate illness. It offers a wide variety of patients, a mix of common and uncommon disorders, a practice based in growth and development, and the possibility to make a real difference in the lives of patients and their families.

> Smooth transition.

> Motherhood and apple pie.

**Example #2.** Like many second-career applicants, this student also felt something meaningful was missing from his career. However, he makes one misstep. In contrasting his future career in psychiatry with his past work in mathematics, he puts down the latter unnecessarily. It is true that making a career change is not easy, but it may sound overblown to characterize it as a monumental achievement.

My pure math activities were enjoyable for themselves, yet I had a growing sense that community service was what gave my life meaning and direction. Did I want to get to the end of my life and answer "What had I done?" with "I proved theorems"? Hoping to use science to help others rather than merely to create more science, I concluded I might be happiest in the long run in medicine, and courageously decided to change careers. So far, medicine has more than fulfilled my expectations as a context to combine the heart and the head. I am particularly intrigued by the doctor-patient relationship, which impresses me as a seamless blend of problem solving, hypothesis-testing, trust-building, and appreciation of the patients' individuality.

> Don't denigrate previous accomplishments.

**Example #3.** This is a well-written paragraph that demonstrates remarkable insight and maturity of thought. The first half of the paragraph is a concise description of his activities during the year off. In the latter half, the applicant shares what he has learned without portraying it as an unprecedented revelation.

After my third year of medical school, I pursued my interest in policy issues studying for a Masters Degree in Public Health at Emory. I spent the year exploring the epidemiology of infectious diseases, options for health care reform, and the empowerment of low-income communities. I learned useful skills in biostatistics and qualitative evaluation, and gained a global perspective on our health care system. At times, however, our discussions of abstract ideas and numbers felt too far removed from the realities of people's lives. I became convinced that debates about health care delivery should be rooted in concrete clinical practice, in the stories of patients and providers. My experience in public health taught me that doctors have a special role in society because they are trusted by patients and respected by policy makers. This combination allows physicians to be potent advocates for their patients and their community.

> Good summary.

> Nice tie-in with his interest in family practice. Clear, concise, and thoughtful.

## Strong Extracurricular/Community Accomplishments

**Example #1.** This applicant has an impressive list of extracurricular activities and achievements. But it is the richness of detail that convinces you that she is diversified and involved in her community.

> Self-motivated, I work vigorously at my research, teaching and patient care. However, it is also very important to me to continue furthering my personal interests, including the creative preparation and presentation of gourmet foods, wreathmaking, and horse training. Especially rewarding is my weekend volunteer work with the Stony Brook Riding Club for the Handicapped that entails rounding up the herd at 6 AM, feeding, grooming, tacking, and assisting the physically and/or mentally disabled riders in any way necessary. Annual CPR organization and instruction to the public brings important education to the community and keeps me abreast of the laymen's current fund of medical knowledge. Additionally, my family background of being the eldest daughter of an architect and a nuclear medicine technologist from Indonesia has led me to a longtime interest in the integration of drawing and science, namely medical illustration. My aspiration is to obtain formal training in illustration technique when my medical education is complete; in the meantime, I hope to continue publishing my drawings and using them in presentations during my residency.

This sentence preempts any concern that the writer's extracurricular activities would interfere with her duties as a resident.

Be careful not to digress; they need a house officer, not an illustrator.

**Example #2.** It is not enough to list your academic accomplishments CV-style. This student highlights the significance of his academic activities in clear, well-organized expository writing.

> Computer consulting work has provided me with close contact with creative researchers in science and medicine. A 2-year thesis project with Dr. Elizabeth Rutter challenged my skills in relational databases, clinical record-keeping systems and exploratory statistical techniques.
>
> In the laboratory of Dr. Jeffrey Greenberg, I applied innovative real-time video microscopy and image processing techniques to fundamental growth and cell-division questions in cell biology. Through my lab work I have developed interests in improving the quality and utility of medical technology for clinical decision making.
>
> I have supplemented medical school by being an active participant in basic biomedical science. In addition to medicine, I am familiar with the tools and vocabulary of modern molecular biology. I read a wide variety of clinical and scientific journals, and use literature searching extensively.

Emphasizes professional skills developed during the project.

Attempts to connect basic science to clinical research.

Applicant seeking research oriented residency skillfully weaves in additional academic activities.

## Poor Academic Performance and Other Blemishes

**Example #1.** There is very little room for excuses in medicine. You either got the job done or you didn't. Unless you have a glaring blemish on your record, excuses will only cause the committee to focus on your weaknesses. In this example the applicant tries to explain why he did not snag more honors. If he had kept his mouth shut, few would have considered this to be a major problem.

On the wards, I found it easy to develop rapport with patients and team members. Ward medicine stimulated my love of scientific inquiry and problem solving. I found enthusiasm, dependability, focused presentations and resilience keys to success. I excelled in medicine clerkships, but my other interests have often required making compromises in pursuing honors in all rotations.

> Risky to make excuses.

## Personal Experiences

**Example #1.**   In some cases, applicants can use general life experiences to become better practitioners. This student, in a dramatic and somewhat risky fashion, indicates that he is able to learn even from painful experiences.

> Unfortunately, not every experience that I had at the University of Rochester was so good, such as the time when I was mugged at gunpoint while walking home from Norton Memorial Hospital on a chilly December evening during my General Surgery rotation. Having been raised in the small town of Brevard, crime was somewhat of a foreign concept to me, as it was just something that I heard mentioned from time to time on the news, thus making this an especially disturbing experience. Although I initially became very cynical and pessimistic, I quickly learned that this type of attitude was not only counterproductive in dealing with life and with patients, but was also very depressing. Eventually, I overcame this frustration, and have learned never to take one's own security, well-being, and confidence for granted. This experience helped me mature as a person, allowing me to understand how frustrating it must be for patients to overcome some of their own physical adversities that have often been inflicted upon them through no fault of their own.

> Be careful with intimate psychological disclosure.

> Makes the effects of a mugging relevant to career.

**Example #2.**   This applicant uses a barebones description of a patient experience to demonstrate her appreciation of the unparalleled access that physicians have to their patients' intimate lives. More detail, however, would give her description some muscle.

> In my second year of medical school I spent one afternoon each week with a primary care physician in San Francisco's Castro district. The practice specialized in caring for HIV-positive homosexual men. In addition to learning about the health care and social issues of this population, the patients and I grew comfortable with each other as I worked to earn their trust. The privilege of health care providers to share difficult times and confidential information with patients was clearly illustrated to me when after an interview a patient remarked, "You know, you're the only woman I've ever talked to about this."

>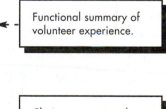
> Functional summary of volunteer experience.

> Choice quote at end adds warmth.

**Example #3.**   This applicant in family medicine makes a basic cultural and human observation through a touching yet humorous experience in an overcrowded Kenyan hospital. The richness of prose is matched by the complexity and maturity of thought behind her observations.

> I found the explanation for my surprising happiness one night in an unusual way. At 3 AM I was called to the wards to admit a young woman

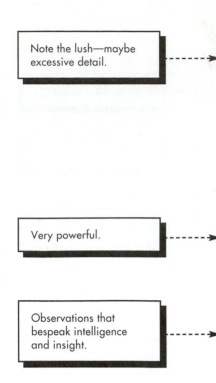

**Note the lush—maybe excessive detail.**

**Very powerful.**

**Observations that bespeak intelligence and insight.**

and arrived to find her comatose, moaning and rocking on her half of a rickety cot. I examined her, hung IV quinine for likely cerebral malaria, did a lumbar puncture, and put down an NG tube as the entire ward of sick women gravely watched the proceedings, their faces eerily illuminated by my penlight, the only source of light. Last to do was the Foley catheter, but try as I might I could not locate the woman's urethra. One of the nurses began to giggle—just a little giggle. I began to giggle. The women on the ward began to smile through their fevers, then chuckle. Soon the entire ward was laughing, great guffaws resounding through that miserable ward. I understood immediately. There was nothing vindictive or belittling in our laughter. On some unspoken group level, really a cultural level, we were pulling together to survive, transcending the almost unbearably hopeless human suffering. No one of us as an individual could hope to escape, but together, as a group, through this laughter—symbolic of some human universal, some common denominator, we stood a chance of retaining our dignity, our perspective, our optimism. Thinking about this moment afterwards, and, indeed, about my whole experience at Mogashi Hospital, I have come to realize the crucial role that cultural constructs—shared belief systems, mutual ways of reacting to circumstances, family, friends, rituals, society—play in an individual's life. . . .

**Example #4.**   Anecdotes about patients are commonly used to highlight an applicant's intelligence and compassion among other traits. Such accounts should, however, be used with discretion. Following is an example that works very well on the first read. However, the story starts to fall apart when you try to understand it on a deeper level. Compare this paragraph to the previous passage; note how much less involved you are in this story. There aren't enough telling details to bring the experience to life. Finally, the "lessons" the writer draws do not seem to unfold from her particular story.

**Writer must have made a connection with the patient, but the message is not clear.**

**Avoid criticizing "all my classes," as the reader probably teaches one.**

During the first week of my outpatient medicine clerkship I met Miss G, a 65-year-old woman who came to the clinic for a routine health assessment. During the course of her evaluation, I obtained a screening mammogram which unfortunately revealed a spiculated mass suggestive of malignancy. For the first time in her life, Miss G faced the possibility of a diagnosis of cancer and realized she must come to terms with her own mortality. For the first time in my life, I found myself looking into the eyes of a patient, trying to be honest and kind while conveying bad news. It was a moment I remember well. I saw Miss G in clinic on several occasions over the ensuing weeks. Although she usually came to see me for health maintenance needs, we invariably turned to her concerns about breast cancer. She approached her fears with remarkable courage and stoicism, finally surrendering to tears of relief when her biopsy was found to be benign. I experienced both a sense of loss and a wonderful feeling of fulfillment when the months in the clinics came to an end. In retrospect, Miss G taught me more about illness, therapy, and what makes a patient "feel better" than I had learned in all of my classes.

## Strong Finishes

**Example #1.** This is an example of a strong finish, somewhat compromised by overuse of the first person singular. The applicant efficiently states his professional and personal goals, highlights notable personal qualities, and sets forth his expectations for residency training—all within five sentences. Unfortunately, each one starts with an "I."

> At UCSF I have experienced tremendous personal growth and have clarified my professional goals. I am committed to developing pragmatic multidisciplinary approaches to improving the quality and delivery of health care in the United States. Personally, I desire to provide compassionate and technically excellent medical care to patients from all walks of life. I will bring to residency energy, enthusiasm, integrity and ability. I expect a challenging, rich environment in which to learn and practice good medicine.

> Very concise.

> Written with conviction and sincerity.

**Example #2.** Many applicants finish with a "ready for anything" type of statement without convincing the reader that they understand what they're getting themselves into. This applicant takes an honest look at the challenges ahead and her ability to meet them. In addition, she balances discussions of her career plans with a glimpse into her personal life. We see how the interplay between work and leisure maintains her balance and stamina.

> I know I have set high goals for myself: clinician, educator, and health advocate. The majority of the time I find working with underserved populations extremely rewarding; however, it can also be emotionally demanding. I have profound admiration for family physicians who have devoted their life to this work. I often grapple with the question of what will enable me to sustain this commitment for a lifetime. The combination of working at an individual level to address health needs and at a more macroscopic level to affect health policy is synergistic for me—each inspires my work in the other. On a personal level, I find my time away from medicine rejuvenating as well. Spending time backpacking, gardening, or being with friends and family enables me to return to work refreshed. Being a physician entails personal sacrifice and dedication, and I am eager to begin the challenge.

> Dose of humility makes applicant seem more human.

> Reality check shows forethought about career plans.

**Example #3.** Female applicants in specialties traditionally dominated by men face special challenges. This surgery applicant injects some machismo into her career discussion/conclusion. Surgery training is often considered a rite of passage. She deals with possible concerns about her commitment to the specialty in the typical surgeon manner—head on. The applicant declares that she can handle anything that surgery training can dish out. In any other specialty, this chest-beating may appear ridiculous. Here her audacity earns respect. It only goes to show that in surgery attitude may be as important as ability.

> The requirements for a surgeon are stringent. Steady hands and a sharp scalpel do not make a surgeon; neither does pure surgical knowledge. Intellectual achievement and community involvement are not enough

Stresses applicant's
determination to
succeed in surgery.

either. A candidate must be equipped with a true sense of commitment to be eligible for a career in surgery. My goals are simple: to learn constantly, so that, in turn, I may teach and heal. The dream of a career in surgery is no longer the naive one sparked first by my father's anecdotes. I am ready to accept the challenges and rigorous demands that accompany a surgeon's life.

# SAMPLE PERSONAL STATEMENTS

In the following pages, we have reproduced some successful personal statements in their entirety, edited only to protect the applicant's identity. Most of the applicants behind these statements matched at top-flight institutions across the country. Once again, commentary is based on the observations of several residency directors, personal statement coaches, and a professional editor.

**Personal Statement #1.** The writer of the following statement left a career in neuroscience research to pursue pediatric neurology. Her statement effectively addresses reasons for delaying medical school, disliking graduate training, and then entering medical school—answering directly the questions a director would have about an older applicant. The essay reads very naturally. Self-effacing humor and enthusiasm for the specialty inflect the essay and compensate for other shortcomings. The essay would have been improved, however, if the applicant had toned down her remarks about her love for the specialty.

When I first entered Oberlin College in 1980 I wanted to go into medicine—it took me 11 years to get there. When I first applied to medical school I thought about pediatric neurology—fortunately, it has not taken me another 11 years. During my third year pediatrics clerkship, I told one of my best friends from college (who is now a primary care attending) that I absolutely loved going to work every day and that I was amazed at how much fun it was to "play with" your patients. Her response was that I could have children of my own and I didn't *need* to go into a field of medicine just to "play with kids." As I continued to love every minute of my other pediatric rotations, I began to realize that of course I didn't *need* to, but that I certainly *could* if it was what I enjoyed the most and what I seemed to do the best.

> **Good motivation.**

When I was in college, I initially put off medicine for entirely the wrong reasons: I hated the competition of the premeds, I could not imagine studying non-stop, and I did not want to stay up all night every 3 to 4 days for years of my life. Instead, I knew that I wanted to study the brain, I had two wonderful role models in my psychobiology career, I got my thesis published, and I headed to graduate school looking forward to a career in neuroscience research. But I feel fortunate now that my 6 years in a graduate program in experimental neuropsychology at UCSD showed me that a career in research by itself was not enough.

> **Appropriate exploration of reasons for entering first career.**

The turning point was deeply personal. My 4-month-old niece was diagnosed with a grade 4 glioblastoma multiforme at the start of my fourth year. I remember sitting in the ICU waiting room at Denver Children's trying to concentrate on a paper related to my dissertation and realizing that what I was studying would never be directly helpful to this beautiful little child or to the rest of my family. It was then that I focused on why I had not been truly satisfied with my graduate experience—something was missing. And I came to realize that what was missing is the very thing that I need and want most from my career—direct application of my work. My personality needs more instant gratification than full-time research was bound to give me. In fact, the only

> **Dramatizes her shift in values.**

gratification that I did seem to be getting routinely in graduate school was through teaching. I loved the interaction with students, the challenge of being an effective communicator, and the sense of responsibility toward the students, all of which are integral parts of being a successful teacher. I received the Distinguished Teacher Award in 1992 and was subsequently appointed to the teaching assistant consultant position responsible for training all the new TAs in the psychology department. Unfortunately, in much of academia, teaching is not as valued a commodity as it should be, and I was constantly made to feel that I was spending "too much time and effort" teaching. As for my research efforts, I am fortunate enough to have experienced the thrill that comes from finding the predicted effects during the final data analysis of my dissertation project, but I know that this thrill would be magnified 10 times if the research had been clinically applicable. I also realized that ultimately I wanted more out of my interaction with patients than having them as research subjects. My experience in medical school has taught me that I was right, there is nothing more rewarding than direct patient care—no matter how challenging it can be. The fact that a career in academic medicine combines the patient care, teaching, and clinical research that I value so much makes me realize how lucky I am to have found this path.

Despite the fact that it was a little disconcerting to turn 30 during my first year of medical school in a class whose mean age was 23, and that it may seem a little harder for me to stay up all night than for my 25-year-old classmates, I have never regretted my path. I feel that the life experience gained from my year as a social worker working with pregnant and parenting teens, and my years in graduate school have contributed immeasurably to my learning of medicine. I knew better during first and second year what was really important—not the grades that I received, but rather how well I could learn to apply that knowledge to a clinical setting. I can also look at the frustrated and angry parents of a sick child and understand a little better what they are going through by applying my experience with my sister and niece.

For a short time during my third year I allowed myself to be steered toward adult neurology by eminent senior faculty members, but I knew there was something in my heart that would not let me make a final career decision until I had experienced child neurology. I went into it with mixed feelings. Another friend who was finishing her pediatrics residency had told me that she had considered doing a neurology fellowship, but thought that it was "too depressing" . . . so she went into oncology instead. I must admit that this scared me. But I knew after only a few days that this was what I was meant to do. I enjoyed every patient interaction I had—the 14-year-old with a static encephalopathy and an intractable seizure disorder, the perfectly normal 4-year-old who came for follow-up after a "bonk" on the head, and the 8-year-old with sudden onset of cranial nerve palsies of still unknown etiology. My learning curve was vertical and I went to sleep every night with Dr. Bruce Silverstein's text on my bed, and then was fortunate enough to have the opportunity to ask him questions in clinic in the morning.

Integrates awards into paragraph on interests.

Light-hearted acknowledgment that medicine is a second career.

Demonstrates how maturity works in applicant's favor.

Humor works surprisingly well here.

Many people have told me how lucky I am to have found a field that I am so enthusiastic about, that to fall so completely in love with something is what everybody hopes for. I knew that day that I went to Toys R Us (post-call) to buy a koosh ball to test visual fields and small plastic toys to test manual dexterity, and the night at 4 AM when I sat in a rocker to console a methadone baby in the nursery before going to bed for that all-important 2 hours' sleep that they were right.

You can chill; we know you like the specialty.

Personal Statement #2. The applicant has done a terrific job making her enthusiasm and convictions visible to us. The introduction is unevenly written, but the decision to launch the essay with a set of reasons for specializing in pediatrics makes the essay focused and direct from the start. In the middle two paragraphs, the applicant's extensive community activities are well described. Overall, the essay is solid and persuasive.

> **The writer scraps a superfluous introduction.**

Of the many contributing factors in my decision to pursue a career in pediatrics, the opportunity for patient education stands out as the most influential. During my clinical clerkships, I discovered many fields to be intriguing and learned from, as well as enjoyed, many aspects of each. It became clear, however, that the rotations providing more patient contact and continuity of care were the most fulfilling. My memories of third-year clerkships are of explaining cardiac catheterization to help allay fears, diagramming reasonable schedules of discharge medications, and discussing puberty with girls beginning their development. Thus, choosing a field became not merely a determination of what I found to be intellectually challenging, but a selection of the role I wished to play in delivering health care to my patients. Pediatrics as a specialty allows the most interaction with patients and their families and affords perhaps the broadest role for the physician, including that of child advocate/social activist, health educator, family friend and role model. Here, colleagues are interested in a patient's adoption history and school performance, and time can be scheduled solely for the purpose of STD teaching.

> **Good motivation.**

In my own educational experiences I have been blessed with supportive teachers who were also excellent role models. I was awarded the opportunity to enter a research laboratory as a high school student largely due to the commitment of a chemistry teacher and the generosity of a pharmacologist. This led to an aspiration to run my own laboratory with a program for future students. In college, a biochemistry professor's encouragement allowed me to pursue an individual project resulting in a publication. Perhaps as a means to reciprocate, I became involved in the local community. I performed the majority of my volunteer work through Alpha Phi Omega, a coeducational service fraternity affiliated with the Boy Scouts of America. Typical activities of the organization were Easter egg hunts for the county's foster children, creating a haunted house every Halloween at the Salvation Army, and providing aid in the aftermath of a local earthquake. Other community-oriented projects included tutoring of Chinatown youths on academic warning. As examples of Asians in college, the tutors also assumed roles of "big siblings" to help the students bridge cultural gaps and to encourage exploration of life opportunities outside the inner city. These activities eventually led me to realize that medicine, with its emphasis on service, would be the more satisfying career for me.

> **"Most rewarding experiences": Good way of organizing paragraph.**

In medical school, I continued my community activities as time permitted. The two most rewarding experiences were that of teaching at a middle school and of organizing a series of talks for fellow pre-professional students. A few classmates and I taught middle schoolers through a program (Med Teach) coordinated by the medical school and the local school district. We had tremendous fun creating lesson plans for 3 classes each week, selecting different topics and styles of

*- teach kids tennis*

*- tutor - Inner city*

*- TA*

presentation for each age group. In addition to short traditional lectures, we often added interactive sessions such as class "Jeopardy" or "pin the organ on the body." One of our lessons on the eye even included group dissection of bovine eyeballs. This interest eventually grew to include the education of fellow classmates. As the community outreach chairperson for the Asian Health Caucus, I wanted medical professionals to learn about the special cultural as well as medical characteristics of the Asian patient (eg, population differences in disease prevalence and drug tolerances). This idea of hosting a single lecture on an Asian health topic was discussed with friends, many of whom voiced wishes for similar talks on other cultural groups. Thus sprouted the day-long Multicultural Health Forum which explored various cultures and their relevant health issues with speakers from different institutions. Moreover, I was able to secure sponsorship from the department of Psychiatry and develop the forum as a credited class with availability to all pre-professional schools including those of pharmacy, nursing, dentistry, and medicine.

> The writer describes a project from start to finish, showing that she can follow through.

I am eager to maintain my interest in teaching, both through patient education and through involvement with medical student training— knowing well the difference an interested resident can make in the medical student experience. Because of this factor, there was never any doubt that I would be best suited for a university based/affiliated pediatrics residency program. I currently anticipate a career in general pediatrics and therefore desire a well-rounded program with strong training in primary care. However, infectious disease and genetics are two areas which I wish to further explore with the option of possible advanced training.

**Personal Statement #3.** This applicant in plastic and reconstructive surgery does a particularly good job detailing research interests without overloading the reader. Note that she rarely has to discuss her interest in plastic surgery in abstract terms—specificity makes this essay work. Through careful attention to her prose, the applicant shows that she cares about her future career in plastics.

As a volunteer anatomy and pathology laboratory instructor, each year I am faced with a new set of students, unpredictable new group dynamics, and ultimately new challenges for presenting material. At times such as these, I truly appreciate the remarkable plasticity of the human mind. A principle taught to me by my own college anatomy instructor, who influenced my career by teaching me *how to teach*, often comes to mind: "Answering a confused student's question with the same words repeatedly is like trying to cut paper by hitting it with a hammer over and over. Instead, trash the hammer and get a pair of scissors," she said, "or start tearing." Through the years, I have learned that effectual communication entails transmission of the understanding that you possess to others, so that they now also understand and are stimulated to think. This requires flexibility and patience, a good understanding and organization of the material, and a high degree of enthusiasm on the part of the teacher. While some of these attributes are inherent in my character, others have been learned and improved upon with every new enterprise.

It is a similar challenge that attracts me to the field of plastic and reconstructive surgery where often there are situations when operative procedures are modified to accommodate a patient's situation. Whether there is a paucity of soft tissue in one area, an abundance of skin in another, or a lack of bone due to destruction or congenital absence, the human body can be made plastic much like the mind modifying the procedures. I welcome and look forward to a lifetime career of meeting these types of challenges creatively in both the adult and pediatric populations, always keeping in mind aesthetics, prognosis, functionality, and the patient's wishes.

Creativity extends to the area of research, which together with teaching, draws me toward a career in academics. To offer a patient an objective list of therapeutic alternatives requires an active hand in contributing to basic and clinical sciences while keeping abreast of the most recent advancements. As an undergraduate in kinesiology at the University of Miami Biomechanics Laboratory, I investigated the recruitment pattern of the medial and lateral gastrocnemius heads in the cat across a continuum of postural and movement demands. To further study pathophysiologic mechanisms of diseases in light of a surgical subspecialty, I completed a Post-Sophomore fellowship with the Florida State Department of Anatomic Pathology, gaining familiarity with frozen biopsy criteria and processing, histologic examination of surgical specimens, special stains, cytologic interpretation, and fresh anatomic dissection during autopsies. Interested in diseases of the musculoskeletal system, I researched a new monoclonal antibody, O13, directed against the p30/32 gene of Ewing's sarcoma and its cross reactivities with other small round blue cell tumors. Possessing a special interest in

Effective use of an anecdote to illustrate a point.

Interesting analogy—plasticity as a parallel between teaching and reconstructive surgery.

Good use of specific details.

pediatric orthopedics, I participated in many of the Toland Hospital for Crippled Children activities over the course of 3 years, including an anesthesia clerkship, contributing to research conducted in the Gait Laboratory, participating in rounds and conferences, and observing a variety of orthopedic surgeries, the majority involving congenital hand abnormalities. It was here that I met Dr. Kathryn Douglass of Baylor University, who introduced me to the notion of approaching a possible hand fellowship from the direction of plastic surgery. Now, with my current interest in plastic and reconstructive surgery, I am presently exploring with Dr. William Schrock at Baylor University the potential of capitalizing upon the angiogenic properties of fibroblast growth factor in the creation of flaps for larger wound coverage secondary to burns or other major trauma.

> The writer's name-dropping is effective because she substantiates the references and explains their significance.

Plasticity, also, is a key virtue during any residency. I am quick to learn new theories and techniques, and able to work well with a wide variety of patient and medical staff personalities. These attributes, coupled with patience and a good sense of humor, have been instrumental in my growth thus far and will continue to be the basic foundation of my philosophy for success in plastic and reconstructive surgery.

**Personal Statement #4.** This very capable statement shows a strong sense of purpose while reviewing several past accomplishments. It offers another example of how to make an applicant's interests appear coherent and consistent.

Jumbled introduction; jumps from fact to fact too quickly.

While growing up in Chicago, I was curious about the city's economic and social segregation, and what could be done to change it. As an English major at Ohio University, I originally intended to teach high school in the inner city, where I felt I might have an impact on education for disadvantaged students. During that time I founded one of the first inner-city Girl Scout troops in Akron and led a troop of 30 girls for 4 years. As the girls began to trust me, they started to ask questions about pregnancy, drugs, and STDs. Although I greatly enjoyed my role as an impromptu health educator, I sensed the futility of providing education without other health resources. Most of these girls received medical care for acute needs only; very few had access to regular primary care. I became increasingly aware of the need for partnership between health education and primary health care. My interest in these issues generated my desire for a career in medicine. I am particularly attracted to Family Practice because it integrates the roles of clinician, educator, and health advocate into the role of physician.

During medical school my primary goal was to develop my clinical skills; however, it was important to me to continue to work with underserved populations to reaffirm my reason for studying medicine. After my first year, I received a scholarship from the Ohio Valley Homelessness Project to study health care access among homeless people.

Impressive achievement, described in detail.

I became acutely aware of the impact of homelessness on health status, and this motivated me to involve other students in this issue. To this end, I helped found a free clinic for homeless people in the 2300 on Main homeless shelter. The Ohio University Students' Homeless Clinic is entirely run by students and volunteer physicians. Since 1991, over 200 students and 30 physicians have provided over 2500 patient visits free of charge. In conjunction with establishing the clinic I also helped develop an elective, currently in its fourth year, on health issues among the homeless. I have remained extremely involved in running the homeless clinic since its inception and currently serve on the Board of Directors. In 1994, I received the Margaret Dawson Award for Outstanding Commitment to Social Action and Social Justice. This is the single award presented at graduation from the School of Public Health.

Sage and succinct.

Working at the clinic constantly reminds me of both my powers and limitations as a future physician. Homeless people have myriad physical, social, and economic factors affecting their health; many have problems far too complex to resolve in a single visit. At first, I was frustrated if patients would come to the clinic requesting moisturizing cream or cough syrup, but were resistant to discussing what I deemed more serious problems—such as substance abuse or hypertension. Eventually, I learned that by first addressing the patient's presenting complaint we could establish trust, which might form the basis for a more

Reinforces primary care philosophy.

continuous relationship. These long-term relationships are what I value most about being a physician. This was affirmed for me in my year-long longitudinal clinic at Swanson Hill Health Center in 1993 as well as during my current longitudinal clinic at the AGH Family Health Center. Through these experiences I have had the opportunity to work with patients on health-related behaviors such as smoking cessation. While trying to change behavior often seems futile or frustrating at a single visit, following patients over a year has shown me the value of incremental change toward healthier lifestyles. The challenges and the rewards of working in this setting reconfirmed my interest in Family Practice.

Dealing with underserved patients' day-to-day medical needs stimulated my interest in studying health care policy on a more global level. As a result, I took a year off between my third and fourth years to pursue a Master's degree in Public Health at Ohio University. My main focus was to examine the factors contributing to the shortage of primary-care physicians in underserved communities. I became convinced that changes in medical education could have an impact on the number of primary care physicians in underserved areas. Along these lines, I was active on a student-faculty committee whose goal was to integrate more primary care and women's health instruction into the curriculum. In addition, through the Department of Family Practice, I am currently researching how medical students' experiences in the homeless clinic affect their choice of a career in primary care and their interest in working with underserved populations. When this work is complete, I intend to submit it for publication.

I know I have set high goals for myself: clinician, educator, and health advocate. The majority of the time I find working with underserved populations extremely rewarding; however, it can also be emotionally demanding. I have profound admiration for family physicians who have devoted their life to this work. I often grapple with the question of what will enable me to sustain this commitment for a lifetime. The combination of working at an individual level to address health needs and at a more macroscopic level to affect health policy is synergistic for me—each inspires my work in the other. On a personal level, I find my time away from medicine rejuvenating as well. Spending time backpacking, gardening, or being with friends and family enables me to return to work refreshed. Being a physician entails personal sacrifice and dedication, and I am eager to begin the challenge.

> The writer makes the year off seem a logical result of her passion for health care, not a deviation in any sense.

> Somewhat weak; let your letter writer mention.

> Personalizes the statement.

*I have met each challenge in my life with hard work and dedication. Whether it was training for a marathon, working full-time while going to school or starting a family, I knew by working hard I would succeed. That's why when I had to take time off during my undergraduate education due to the financial strains of living in New York and starting a family, I knew this would be a momentary delay of achieving my life long goal of becoming a doctor. After my wife and I were able to obtain some financial security, I finished my B.S. in Physiology at the University of Arizona and was accepted into St. Lucas University School of Medicine.*

*St. Lucas University is located on the beautiful island of St. Kitts in the British West Indies. Most of the classes are taught by retired professors from U.S. medical schools. Besides the excellent education I received, the life experiences my wife and I gained living in a foreign country without the amenities of the U.S. were priceless. We will never forget washing our clothes in the sink or searching for propane gas to cook with on our stove.*

*I finished my Basic Sciences with a 3.96 GPA. I went on to score a 246/95 on the USMLE Step 1. My high score placed me at Douglas Medical Center (DMC) in Fresno, California for all of my clinical rotations. DMC is an excellent county hospital affiliated with University Hospital School of Medicine which accepts the best students from St. Lucas University into its clerkship program. DMC provided me with a well-rounded clinical experience and prepared me well for the USMLE Step 2, which I scored a 255/98 on. Also, during my Surgery core rotation my beautiful baby girl was born.*

*Although I have found all my clinical rotations interesting, I experienced the most excitement from my time in Anesthesia. Anesthesia offers me the opportunity to integrate my basic science knowledge with clincial care. In no other rotation did I have the hands on application of basic sciences, every OR case was a mini-experiment in pharmacology and physiology. The fast pace and the constant demand for rapid clear thinking made my time in Anesthesia nothing but exhilarating. My rotation also showed me the various duties of the Anesthesiologist beyond the OR and the integral part they play in Labor and Delivery, the Emergency Room, the Intensive Care Unit and in the management of pain.*

*On a personal level, I find my time away from medicine rejuvenating as well. Spending time running, mountain biking, surfing, and being with my wife and daughter enables me to return to work refreshed.*

*My career goal is to enter a university based Anesthesiology program. I believe my strong science knowledge base, clinical experience and ability to make quick decisions are well suited for Anesthesiology. I am highly detailed-oriented and enjoy being part of a cohesive medical care team. I look forward to the education, practice and research opportunities available in Anesthesiology.*

---

[1] Reproduced, with permission, from the Medschool.com Community website (http://students.medschool.com).

*During medical school I became involved in research with Dr. Z. in the Department of Anatomy and Neurobiology at Medical State University. I utilized the skills I had obtained through my bachelor's degree in visual arts toward our project. The manual dexterity I acquired through artwork allowed me ease in performing microscopic, stereotaxic surgeries; my work with chemistry in photographic development proved useful in immunohistochemical staining of our injection sites; and my illustrative abilities were applied in mapping the axonal projections of the nuclei. My background in art has provided me a breadth of knowledge that enriches my approach to medicine. I continue in my tradition of challenging myself in new areas: entering medicine with a background in art, presenting and publishing research, and now endeavoring to become a dermatologist.*

*Dermatology is the field in which many of my interests and skills converge. The pattern, texture, and color of artwork are discussed in a similar manner as skin pathology is described. I am confident in my ability to appreciate and interpret the visual manifestation of disease. I enjoy creating a precise image of primary and secondary lesions in order to develop a thorough and accurate differential diagnosis.*

*Comprehension of histopathology is essential to the study of dermatology. Through my prior work in a surgical pathology lab and experience performing biopsies in my dermatology rotations, I have acquired an appreciation of the processes involved in and the necessity of obtaining adequate samples of tissue for diagnosis and treatment. I have refined my procedural skills through my experience in microscopic surgery and in suturing Mohs repairs.*

*As with most areas of medicine, relating to patients with understanding and empathy is a priority in dermatology. I have developed my interpersonal skills by interacting with a variety of people through my study of art, my residence abroad within a different culture, and my current work in medicine. Open communication with others has come with ease. I value the mutual respect and trust that develops between physician and patient; I witness the healing effect that such a relationship has in treating patients.*

*As a field that continuously changes through medical and technological advances, dermatology encourages the ability to engage in research. Having completed a study observing trends in basal cell carcinoma in an individual surgery practice, I am currently coauthoring a chapter on different types of skin cancer to be published in a medical journal designed for general practitioners. I anticipate continuing in research throughout residency and my career in academic dermatology.*

*One of my greatest motivations in studying medicine is the opportunity to study and learn throughout my career. My introduction to dermatology in medical school generated great interest and a desire to learn much more about its practice and new developments. I appreciate the expanse of material involved and knowledge yet to acquire in the study of dermatology.*

*Dermatology is a field in which I can continue to challenge myself. Through my rotations in surgery and general dermatology, I have discovered that it is the field of medicine for which I am best suited. I eagerly anticipate engaging in and contributing to the study of the skin and its manifestation of disease. My studies in art and involvement in research have enriched my medical education and will continue to provide a unique and enlightened approach to the practice of dermatology.*

---

[2]Reproduced, with permission, from the Medschool.com Community website (http://students.medschool.com).

*During my junior year at UCLA, I became certified as an emergency medical technician (EMT), a decision that had a profound effect on my life. I was subsequently hired by UCLA Emergency Medical Services (EMS) and staffed the campus ambulance, serving as a first responder for all medical aid calls on the UCLA campus and neighboring communities. There was a tremendous sense of responsibility in being the first medical provider on scene to assess and provide treatment for potentially unstable patients in unpredictable environments. In addition to cementing my desire to attend medical school, my experience with UCLA EMS introduced me to the field of emergency medicine.*

*At the completion of my first year of medical school, I was awarded the Student Research Committee Fellowship. This fellowship supported a research project designed to evaluate the safety and efficacy of external cardiac pacing of patients with symptomatic bradycardia by paramedics in the pre-hospital setting. This two-and-a-half year project was supervised by the Medical Director of the San Francisco Fire Department. The data demonstrated a trend toward increased survival among patients treated with external cardiac pacing compared to those treated with conventional therapy alone. Based upon this data, the State of California Emergency Medical Services Commission approved external cardiac pacing as first-line therapy for this patient population, permitting EMS providers throughout the State to perform this procedure.*

*Throughout medical school, I was aware of my interest in emergency medicine, but made a conscious effort not to prematurely exclude other specialties. I thought I might find one clerkship to stand out among them all, calling me to devote my life to it. Instead, I found them all incredibly challenging and fulfilling, particularly those experiences requiring immediate decisions to be made, procedures to be performed, and most of all, trips to the emergency department. My greatest sense of achievement, regardless of the clerkship, was when I was caring for patients with an acute illness, exacerbation of a chronic disease, or a traumatic injury.*

*I am eager to begin my residency training and look forward to expanding my knowledge base, becoming more adept in assessment, diagnosis, and treatment in the acute setting, and gaining the experience necessary to become a well-rounded, confident physician. I hope to train in a facility with a culturally diverse patient population, a broad variety of trauma, medical illness, pediatric emergency experience, EMS exposure, and clinical research opportunities. In addition to supporting my growth as a physician, I want to train at a program that supports my development outside the hospital, encouraging continued participation in my personal interests, such as exercising, camping, and traveling.*

*My long-term goals include attending in a high-acuity, academically oriented, Level 1 trauma center that conducts high-quality clincial research. I am also interested in pursuing a fellowship in emergency medical services to enhance my ability to promote quality prehospital care. My understanding of the field of emergency medicine has vastly matured from my days as a EMT. I now realize that the realm of the emergency physician extends well beyond the back of an ambulance or the entrance to a hospital. Emergency physicians are regularly faced with the entire spectrum of medical and surgical disease, requiring immense skill, diagnostic acumen, and empathy for both the frightened patient and concerned family members. In this era of managed care and cost containment, emergency physicians must be conservative in their diagnostic evaluations, yet remain aggressive in their pursuit of excluding acutely life-threatening illnesses. More importantly, emergency physicians serve as powerful patient advocates and valuable liaisons between the medical community and general public.*

*I feel I have proven myself capable of compassionate, competent care during my clinical years and have no doubt that I will greatly benefit from residency training in emergency medicine. I eagerly await the next phase of my education and welcome the challenges and excitement it will bring.*

---

[3]Reproduced, with permission, from the Medschool.com Community website (http://students.medschool.com).

*Although I started medical school with an inclination toward primary care, my choice of family medicine was not a foregone conclusion. I have considered many areas of specialty throughout my medical school experiences, but I keep returning to family medicine as the best match for my vocational goals and personality. Family medicine attracts me for several reasons. First, family medicine allows me to treat a wide variety of patient populations and illnesses. My medical school training and extracurricular interactions have given me the opportunity to serve all age groups, from infants to the elderly. I love children and gave serious thought to a career in pediatrics. Yet I also enjoy aspects of orthopedics, obstetrics, psychiatry, and geriatric care. I feel that family medicine offers me the most interesting spectrum of patient care. Although some may view this variety as a daunting challenge, I see it as a constant spark of excitement in the practice of medicine.*

*I also find family medicine attractive because of its role in small communities. Unlike other medical specialties, family medicine affords me the opportunity to live and serve in a small town. I feel that a family doctor can fill an important need in small and often under served communities. I look forward to offering quality, up-to-date medical care in a setting where my patients and I interact on a first name basis and where I can offer treatment based on perhaps a more intimate knowledge of my patients' backgrounds. I found this to be true during my family medicine clerkship in rural Idaho as a fourth year medical student. My experience in Idaho convinced me that I could enjoy serving as a family doctor in a small community. On a more personal level, a small community is a great environment for raising a family, and my wife and I would like our children to grow up in such an environment.*

*I also feel that family medicine has a unique and vital role in educating families and providing preventative care. As I teach parents about developmental milestones, immunizations, give anticipatory guidance, and prescribe treatments for childhood illnesses, I do more than treat one sick child. As I teach adults principles of healthy diet and exercise, I do more than avert heart disease. Such education has the potential to help generations live healthy lives. Age-appropriate screening and counseling are other important roles I look forward to as a family doctor.*

*Several influential family practitioners in my life have given me additional impetus for choosing family medicine myself. Dr. W. not only brought me into the world, but he also delivered and continued to care for my twin brother and four other brothers and sisters over the years. Several years later, he was able to deliver my sister's children as well. Of course this scenario is not always possible in today's transient society where people change insurance plans and doctors frequently. However, the opportunity for this kind of long-term interaction with families seems to still exist in instances in family medicine. As a teenager my family doctor became a trusted friend and respected adult figure in my life. Dr. M. was able to relate to my teenage issues and treated me with appropriate respect. He showed me that a doctor can have a positive influence on a patient's life far beyond traditional medical cures.*

*Years ago, I was stymied as I tried to select an undergraduate course of study that would best help me in a medical career. I consulted several medical professionals and asked their opinions as to which major would best help me in a medical practice. Many respected family practitioners advised me to major in business so that I could better manage my own family practice someday and assured me that such an education would benefit me in any type of practice. They also felt that choosing a major outside the basic science curriculum (which I would still be learning as a prerequisite for medical school) could only enrich and broaden my education. Now that I have decided upon family practice, I am grateful for their advice and look forward to applying some of the business fundamentals I learned in my own practice of medicine.*

*Finally, family practice appeals to me because of its focus on the family unit. My family—my beautiful wife and two children, as well as extended family—is the most important thing in my life. I want to become the type of doctor that my own children, wife, mother, and grandmother would feel comfortable and confident turning to for medical care.*

---

[4]Reproduced, with permission, from the Medschool.com Community website (http://students.medschool.com).

*"Far and away the best prize that life offers is the chance to work hard at work worth doing."—Theodore Roosevelt*

*My parents carefully measured out their wisdom like coffee grounds, shake hands firmly . . . look everyone in the eyes . . . never complain . . . work harder . . . smile and enjoy . . . always do the right thing. The experience of living has been the water that percolates through these lessons, ultimately defining my cardinal principles of work and life.*

*Passion, beneficence, and excellence are fundamental to these principles and drive my pursuit of general surgery. Passion. Everyday I strive to deserve the privilege of practicing surgery. From my earliest research experiences with cardiac surgery in dogs, I have aspired to learn enough, work enough, and care enough to earn the trust of my future patients and colleagues.*

*This passion is my sustaining force. It is the excitement that kept me up through four emergency appendectomies starting at midnight. It is the calm that steadied my hand to insert a chest tube and drop a central line at a 4 AM trauma. It is the sympathy that gave me patience to hear Mr. H's story detailing each evening's mighty struggle to stuff a volleyball-sized hernia back into his abdomen for 22 years before coming in for surgery.*

*This passion motivates me to be a great surgeon. Beneficence. I am devoted to improving the way things work, I believe that basic scientific research and medical education are essential for enhanced patient care. However, administrational efforts outside the immediate realm of medicine are also important to forging advancements in health care. After identifying a deficit in funding of student research, I developed a proposal for an endowed fellowship for scientific investigation. Resulting from a combination of numerous meetings, letters, and a big piece of my heart, the alumni trustees, medical center administrators, and university financiers agreed to endow over half a million dollars for a fellowship to support medical student research. This fellowship is funded for perpetuity and provides $25000 to one student annually to pursue independent research. The first fellowship was awarded this past spring to a promising second-year who wants to cure cancer. Whether or not she achieves her goal, it is the spirit and talent of thousands of students and scientists like her that impel progress in medical science. My desire and ability to produce tangible improvements will benefit the field of general surgery.*

*Excellence. I am always searching for ways to improve myself as a human being and as a surgeon. Because a problem-based curriculum afforded a flexible schedule, I was able to regularly participate in service projects, most often visiting elementary schools to discuss safe sex and drugs with high-risk children. Frequently, later in the evenings, I helped treat sexually transmitted diseases at an indigent clinic.*

*I chose to explore fields related to a career in surgery through a year of independent research. By putting my head down to get through the daily grind, I overcame the obstacles of gel exposure snafus, cell culture contamination, and editing for publication, to be productive in basic and clinical projects. My achievements in this previously unfamiliar territory—I was a philosophy major in college—have given me the experience, confidence, and motivation to support research as I move onto my next stage of training.*

*This commitment to self-improvement maximizes my abilities and opportunities. By remaining true to my cardinal principles I will enthusiastically strive towards, and hopefully lead, the promotion of patient care as a surgeon. Benefiting from my experiences and equipped with knowledge, effort, and spirit, I am prepared to continue such work worth doing.*

---

[5]Reproduced, with permission, from the Medschool.com Community website (http://students.medschool.com).

*Choosing a specialty in medicine, like medical school in general, is a unique experience that will make a tremendous impact on the rest of your personal and professional life. Many students are dead set on specific careers before they even make their first shaky incision in gross anatomy. Others think they know which field they ultimately want to pursue, only to discover later on that everything about their chosen specialty disagrees with them. Then there are students like me, who go to medical school armed with the knowledge that ultimately they'll become doctors, but not really knowing which kind.*

*When I began my medical education, I was honestly surprised to learn that many of my new classmates were already committed to specific paths, some of them with extensive research and experience in their fields of choice. My older brother, who changed his mind at least three times before he applied for residency, had advised me to wait until the clinical years so that I could make an informed choice and that had been my plan from the beginning. But as more and more of my friends began narrowing down their choices in the first two years of school, my plan to wait to make a decision suddenly felt like procrastination. Nevertherless, with limited clinical exposure and plenty of studying to keep me busy, I resigned myself to following my brother's advice and to wait until my third year.*

*Making the abrupt shift from bookworm to third-year clinical clerk, was both a nerve-wracking and exciting prospect. Although we had discussed the doctor-patient relationship and the art of medicine during the first two years of school, the opportunities to practice those concepts were few and far between. Interviewing patients for an hour once a week, didn't seem like a realistic picture of things to come (it wasn't). I was nervous about balancing a schedule that I knew would be hectic, being responsible for patients while trying to read about diagnosis, pathophysiology, and treatment. Mostly, I was excited that I'd finally have the chance to learn how to care for people and to explore possible future careers. My introduction to clinical medicine was cut short though. That fall, my mother was scheduled for extensive spinal surgery in an effort to relieve years of discomfort, and I was granted a leave of absence by the school and returned to Los Angeles to be with her for the next six months. When I returned in the winter to begin my clerkships, I realized that it was impossible to finish all the necessary requirements in time to graduate in 1999 and I became a member of the class of 2000.*

*In retrospect, taking the extra time was a serendipitous blessing in disguise. It allowed me to objectively approach the clinical clerkships without rushing to make a career decision. As I rotated through the various specialties, I began to get a better understanding of what I found interesting. Initially, radiology was one field that intrigued me, combining technology and intuition to clarify disease pathology. I signed up for electives and became involved in research, hoping to further stoke my interest and solidify my desire to possibly pursue radiology as a career. Instead, it had the opposite effect. I quickly realized that although I found the images and technology amazing, I sorely missed the direct one-to-one patient contact that we had talked about during the first two years and that we had been introduced to during the third year.*

*People often say that the lessons learned along the way are what make a journey worthwhile, that the opportunities to gain insight and acquire knowledge can be easily missed if you simply focus on traveling from point A to point B. It is this idea that embodies my experiences in medical school and which has led me to my decision to pursue internal medicine as a career. What I've realized is that the things I find most rewarding are developing relationships with patients and being in an environment that fosters continuity of care. Caring for patients from admission to discharge and following up long term to provide for their healthcare needs is what I ultimately want to base my career as a physician upon. Everyone who goes to medical school has unique experiences that lead them to discover their own personal niches. To me, internal medicine covers a wide spectrum of disease pathology while allowing personal relationships to develop with patients, offering the ideal blend of academic challenge and personal fulfillment. In this way, I can share in the lessons learned from other people's journeys while I continue on my own.*

[6]Reproduced, with permission, from the Medschool.com Community website (http://students.medschool.com).

*During a clerkship in my third year of medical school in my hometown of St. Louis, I was struck by a comment made by a nurse one morning before rounds. She recognized my name as being the same as two previous physicians who cared for her and her family. These physicians were my grandfather and great grandfather. She then went on to tell me that my great grandfather had delivered her, and that my grandfather cared for her during her childhood at his office. What moved me most by what she said was how tangible my relationship to my grandfather had become, and the very meaningful impact they had made on this nurse's life. I chose to go into medicine during college on my own accord, yet the fact that I have two previous family members who were a part of this profession gives me a profound sense of integrity and responsibility.*

*Throughout my schooling, working directly with people has always interested me. My experience while attending Loyola University in New Orleans, where I worked as a health assistant for two years, helped me to realize that I would succeed in medicine. A month long trip during my senior year of college to a village in Nicaragua challenged my ability to communicate and work with people, and solidified even more my desire to study medicine. Multiple involvement during medical school, such as coordinating a student run clinic on several Saturdays, supported my interest in primary care, and at the same time fostered leadership skills and a better sense of team spirit.*

*My rotation in internal medicine at a Veterans Administration hospital, the first of my third year clerkships, initiated a desire to pursue the specialty of internal medicine. I was exposed to patients with conditions ranging from asthma to resistant HIV, which I found to be intellectually challenging and professionally fulfilling. Later in the course of my third year, my exposure to pediatrics paralleled my experience in internal medicine, and my learning cue took off even more. Now I find myself using the medical literature more frequently to support my rising interests. I find clinic to be a rewarding interaction, and a wonderful chance to counsel parents/guardians.*

*My interest in combined internal medicine and pediatrics as a specialty solidified at the end of my third year of medical school. Primary care is my interest. Seeing and helping patients of a wide age range and of various clinical presentations is what I want to focus on. My enthusiasm for internal medicine and pediatrics is both complementary and synergistic. I intend to take full advantage of the training offered and become an extremely competent, well trained and respected physician. In short, I want to be a resource for my patients and a source of appropriate medical care. The variety of patients in this setting draws me toward this field, and will keep me continually interested and enthusiastic throughout the course of my career. The fact that I will comprehensively train in treating children and adults alike compels me to pursue internal medicine/pediatrics.*

*The bridge and relationship between the two areas, in my perception, are well connected. In my student experience, both internal medicine and pediatrics hold a common approach to patients. Their corresponding knowledge funds are both diverse and comprehensive. I look forward to being able to employ that knowledge competently and effectively throughout the course of my career.*

[7]Reproduced, with permission, from the Medschool.com Community website (http://students.medschool.com).

Among many other things I have learned in medical school, I have come to the opinion that the role people assume in the somewhat conservative field of medicine involves wearing a relatively thick professional mask. This is not necessarily negative, as there is no denying that an air of competence and compassion is certainly inspiring to patients. However, perhaps in part because I have never been a particularly accomplished actor myself, I find it all the more interesting when that mask is taken off and the true self emerges through all the layers of professionalism. When one truly enjoys his job, the most fun and energetic part of his personality emerges. When a patient presents with a rare and interesting disease, or when there is a captivating diagnostic problem, physicians who love their jobs bring their full intellect and attention to bear. Then, amazingly, all the layers of formality and pride are peeled away to reveal an enthusiasm to solve the problem and share their knowledge and excitement, which I find extremely infectious. In that moment when a diagnostic test is performed, or when a novel scientific result is on the brink of revealing itself, we are all transformed into a curious child all over again, whether we are students, attendings, or Nobel laureates.

I have chosen neurology as a specialty because it is a field that fascinates me to that point of enthusiasm—an enthusiasm that I wish to share with my patients, future colleagues, and students. I believe that the central nervous system has so much intrinsic interest that it draws a higher proportion of physicians who are genuinely captivated by their field. An important benefit from this is that it provides for the opportunity to work with others with similar enthusiasm, enabling a more enjoyable and educational experience. The clinical work is interesting and satisfying to me because of the close association of findings on the history and physical exam with the lesion location and etiology. I also find some of the more subtle cognitive deficits from brain pathology to be extremely interesting, shedding light on the function of arguably the most important, complex, and uniquely human organ of the body.

I feel that neurology remains a final frontier of biomedicine, with many clinical and scientific truths yet to be unraveled and translated for the benefit of human health and knowledge. In an era when molecular genetic approaches are rapidly revolutionizing the field of medicine, neurology stands poised to gain significant therapeutic benefit, as many cerebral disorders appear beyond our present ability to cure. It is especially fulfilling for me to be able to offer help in these areas where it is sorely needed, and I anticipate a day when we have the power to prevent or cure intractable diseases like ALS or Alzheimer's disease as research efforts from the Decade of the Brain yield fruit. During my third year of medical school, I had the exciting opportunity to work on a basic problem in neurophysiology at the National Institutes of Health with a fellowship from the Howard Hughes Medical Institute. From my experience at the NIH, I have gained an enormous appreciation for the scientific efforts in elucidating the workings of the nervous system and the process involved in finding treatments for specific disorders. I was able to meet very accomplished physicians in the research arena who serve as my role models. The experience has been instrumental in shaping my career aspirations to pursue a biomedical research career, which appeals to the creative side of my personality. In addition to medical and scientific impact, neurology and neuroscience are fields whose questions have far-reaching implications for apparently unrelated fields such as religion and philosophy. By providing insights into mechanisms of behavior and consciousness, it addresses critical questions related to our essential humanity, which I find extremely intellectually stimulating.

I hope that with my sincere passion for the field, a diligent work ethic, and a good-natured team attitude, I will be able to help alleviate suffering from neurologic disease and simultaneously learn about how our minds work. For the future, I hope to be a part of the forefront of our advancing understanding of the neurological sciences and use that knowledge to heal our patients and train others interested in the field. For these reasons, I have chosen to specialize in neurology with an eventual goal of practicing, teaching, and conducting research at an academic hospital.

---

[8] Reproduced, with permission, from the Medschool.com Community website (http://students.medschool.com).

## Personal Statement Samples: Neurosurgery[9]

*Very few matriculating medical students can realistically determine their future career choices. We all enter with the altruistic goals of becoming caring physicians and making a significant contribution to medicine. As lay persons, we do not grasp the breadth of medicine and often are unaware of its specialization. I myself come from a medical family background and therefore had a somewhat greater exposure to medicine, but I was in no way qualified upon entering medical school to conclude on a career in a particular specialty. In spite of this, I always entertained the notion of becoming a neurosurgeon.*

*The central nervous system represented to me the most intriguing and complex human organ system. During my first two medical school years, I was fascinated by the study of the central nervous system including its intricate three dimensional anatomy, physiology, and pathology. During my third year of medical school, I gravitated towards the surgical specialties. I had the opportunity to become a member of the University of Mississippi neurosurgical team and participate in many neurosurgical procedures; an experience that I greatly enjoyed. The meticulous surgeries and the application of intricate anatomical knowledge and physiology markedly impressed me. Neurosurgery offers the challenge of not merely maintaining a patient's life, but of sustaining their spirit, intelligence, and personality. Unlike almost any other field, neurosurgery deals with the elements that contribute to our consciousness and make us human. These experiences led to the coalescence of my decision to pursue a career in neurosurgery.*

*My professional goals include the completion of a comprehensive neurosurgical residency training in conjunction with basic science research experience and subsequently pursuing a career in academic neurosurgery. The academic discourse and the intellectual stimulation afforded in an academic environment are appealing as well as the opportunity to participate in the endeavor of furthering the scope of our knowledge. I will strive to follow the clinician/scientist model that I admire and I hope to develop a research program complementary to my clinical interests. On my part, I bring the desire to work hard, participate actively in my own education, and a deep commitment to make a positive contribution to my residency program and neurosurgery.*

*I believe that my credentials to pursue a career in neurosurgery include my strong academic background. I began my undergraduate education at Clemson University where I was elected to the Phi Eta Sigma Freshman Honor Society before transferring to Georgia Tech University because of my desire to be closer to my family secondary to an illness in the family. At Georgia Tech University, I was elected to the Phi Beta Kappa Honor Society and received the College of Liberal Arts and Sciences (CLAS) Outstanding Scholar Award, an award conferred on the graduating CLAS student with the highest grade point average. At the University of Mississippi School of Medicine, I was awarded the Board of Trustees Academic Scholarship and continued my strong academic performance. Additionally, I was honored with the Basic Science Research Scholarship on the basis of an original research proposal involving the synaptic integration and information processing carried out in a single nerve cell. The research culminated in a poster presentation at the Eastern Student Research Forum. I have used that experience to pursue neurosurgical research relating to spinal cord injury that is currently in progress.*

*Aside from academics, I have been active in the Mississippi Medical Association and have visited that state capital on several occasions to observe and participate in the lobbying process. Currently, I am serving on the Mississippi Medical Association's Public Relations Council and participating in the planning of programs designed to increase membership in our professional medical associations and raise physician awareness concerning current medically related political issues in the rapidly changing managed care market. For recreation, I am an active participant in pickup basketball games and make an effort to weightlift on a consistent basis. I have also maintained an interest in the rapidly growing area of the Internet and recently published an article concerning the Internet's medical applications. I am also currently in the process of constructing a homepage for the University of Mississippi's Neurosurgery Department.*

[9]Reproduced, with permission, from the Medschool.com Community website (http://students.medschool.com).

# Personal Statement Samples: Obstetrics and Gynecology[10]

*While my path to becoming a physician has always been a straight one, my interest in the field of obstetrics and gynecology has come full circle. During vacations from college, I worked in the office of an obstetrician-gynecologist in Washington, DC. Excited by the breadth of patients that he saw, I was also impressed by the surgical nature of the field. Thus, I began medical school believing I would one day be an obstetrician-gynecologist. During my first two years of medical school, however, I drifted from this belief and considered the areas of medicine and pediatrics. However, the experiences of my third year helped me to better focus my interests. While I was impressed with the thought processes involved in the evaluation of patients during my medicine rotation, I was often frustrated by the inability to physically do something to help. During my pediatrics rotation, I was amazed by the young body's ability to heal, although I often felt this healing had less to do with the medical team than with the body's natural defenses. The resiliency of my patients, coupled with the opportunity to practice preventative medicine and primary care, initially left me thinking I would enter the field of pediatrics. I began obstetrics and gynecology excited to see babies delivered, but otherwise completely naïve that this was my calling. After just a short time on the rotation, I found myself feeling not obligated to read at home, but excited to learn more about the problems I had faced that day. As in pediatrics, it was refreshing to see a generally young, healthy patient population. However, unlike in pediatrics, in obstetrics and gynecology there was often the opportunity to physically do something that would lead to beneficial outcomes. I look forward to the opportunities to combine prevention and treatment strategies to keep my patients healthy.*

*I see my career occupied not just with medicine, but with influence in healthcare policy and management. During medical school, I have come to appreciate the quantity and complexity of healthcare issues today. I realize that as a medical student and resident I must focus on learning the facts and skills needed to be a successful clinician, but I also believe that knowledge of and participation in the vast number of healthcare decisions being made each day is imperative for a clinician. For this reason, I plan to constantly continue my education, both in the professional setting and by earning a degree in either public policy or business administration. With knowledge and credentials, I will become actively involved in creating and implementing healthcare policy that focuses on the needs of patients rather than of insurance companies or administrators.*

*I have always had an interest in education and community outreach, and my goal is to make a difference in the policies of the healthcare system. Access to healthcare in rural and urban communities is a serious problem that our nation faces, and I feel obligated to use my knowledge and background to help, whether on a local or national level. My desire to improve communities in need is long-standing. An important influence on this interest began with my high school sociology teacher and friend, Mr. C. Progressive in his requirement of 20 community service hours per semester, he stressed the importance of reaching out to others. Because of his hands-on approach, I learned about my responsibility to help others. Unfortunately, Mr. C died of complications arising from AIDS in February 1994. At his memorial service, a speaker asked the mourners to look around the crowded auditorium full of people whose lives Mr. C had touched, a group that represented just a fraction of the whole. The speaker reminded us that if each of us could touch just one other person in the same way, and that person would touch one more person, and so on, the memory of Mr. C would never be lost. I choose medicine as my way to impart knowledge, to give hope, and to touch others with love and understanding.*

---

[10]Reproduced, with permission, from the Medschool.com Community website (http://students.medschool.com).

## Personal Statement Samples: Ophthalmology[11]

*A person who feels a specific calling in his life is a fortunate person. While we never know what the future may hold for us, having a definite direction in which to travel is a real blessing and a rare occurrence. My calling to pursue a career in ophthalmology came after 3 years of dedication to studying the human body, interacting with patients, and "trying on" various medical specialties in my third year of rotations. My interest in the eye, however, began in my second year during the ophthalmology section of the mechanisms of disease class. I found the intricacy and vastly varied pathology of the visual system to be fascinating. Even more interesting was the small amount of clinical exposure to ophthalmology in our third year curriculum. Except for four afternoons spent in ophthalmologists clinic during the general practice clerkship (I am convinced this rotation made more ophthalmologists than general practitioners), the eye was not discussed much, but I thirsted for more knowledge in this area.*

*My firsthand experience with ophthalmology came under the guidance of a second year ophthalmology resident, whom I greatly respect spiritually, personally, and professionally. I met him at a church youth-group function, and he invited me to visit the triage area of the emergency department. I spent a day in the emergency room with him where he showed me patient after patient, each case more interesting than the one before. The patients were very concerned about their vision. As he went though the general exam with me, pointing out the varying pathology, he calmed each patient by explaining the details of their illness and treatment. After watching him during a few more visits to the ER, I knew I wanted to be this type of physician. Furthermore, after a day in the OR with an attending physician and a few discussions with my student advisors, I knew I wanted to treat these types of patients.*

*During medical school, my family and friends, who remain a very important part of my life, complemented my influences in the medical field by providing support and fellowship in a non-academic arena. My mother, a school psychologist, and my father, a retired USAF pilot, continue to provide counsel from my hometown in Florida. My brother, a lawyer (in a firm that represents doctors and hospitals), also encourages me from his home in Florida. Following their example I have been able to establish a strong work ethic and moral basis from which to guide my career. I have also been fortunate enough to pass along my experiences and advice to the youth at my church during church functions, including the annual youth choir trip. Throughout medical school, I believe I have learned the value of hard work, punctuality, discipline, knowledge, and a good attitude. These values are contagious, and I look forward to bringing them to whatever work environment I encounter.*

*Ophthalmology contains all of what I love about the medical profession; medicine, surgery, treatment of both the old and the young, primary care, and specialized procedures. Ophthalmology is also a dynamic field, with frequent new advances in preserving or improving people's vision. I will enjoy the challenge of keeping up with new developments and will take satisfaction in contributing to that growth. Having a calling that will grant me the opportunity to positively impact people's eyesight and health while offering them compassion during a stressful time will be a rewarding experience and a rich personal blessing.*

---

[11]Reproduced, with permission, from the Medschool.com Community website (http://students.medschool.com).

# Personal Statement Samples: Orthopedic Surgery[12]

Running has been an integral part of my life since high school when I became involved in cross-country and track. During college and medical school I have continued running and have completed several road races and two triathlons. Running has taught me the value of patience, dedication, and perseverance; provided an outlet for stress; and kept me physically and mentally fit. It was also through running that I began to appreciate the importance of the musculoskeletal system. I would periodically sustain various sports-related injuries, which led to my first exposure to the field of orthopedic surgery.

While I believe the traits I developed as a runner prepared me for the rigors of surgery, my interest in orthopedic surgery stems from my fascination with the effects of structure on function. From fashioning various creations out of Legos as a child to constructing electronic circuits and building off-road remote control cars as an adolescent, I have always enjoyed learning about how things work. As a young teen I built a cabin with my cousin and uncle. I was enthralled during each step of the process; drafting the plans, setting the foundation, constructing the walls, laying the roof, and weatherproofing the exterior.

The opportunity to visualize and mentally construct objects in three dimensions combined with an interest in how the building blocks of life are put together attracted me to organic chemistry and biochemistry. In these courses I learned how minor changes in molecular structure could have drastic effects on chemical properties. While exploring the structure and function of cells and molecules through research, I became increasingly fascinated with the anatomy and physiology of the human body. During medical school, I conducted research using a rat model to investigate the effects of interleukin-10 on inflammation associated with venous thrombosis. This experience allowed me to gain familiarity with operating on rats under a low power microscope, examining and preparing surgical specimens, and taking gross and histologic photographs. I particularly enjoyed operating on the rats, which enhanced my interest in surgery.

In addition to acquiring new knowledge via research, I also enjoy sharing knowledge with others through teaching. My mentors demonstrated time and time again how the combination of hard work and talent could allow a person to reach his or her fullest potential. My father, one of my greatest mentors as well as a physician, has shown me that happiness and tremendous personal satisfaction can be acquired by making a difference in patients' lives. It is these principles as well as factual concepts that I strive to share with students. As a senior in college I helped other prospective medical students prepare for the MCAT by teaching classes for KAPLAN Educational Centers. In the year before I began medical school, I was a teaching assistant for an honors organic chemistry laboratory and discussion group.

In medical school I have experienced tremendous personal growth and have focused my career objectives. Key elements that I have used to achieve continued success include maintaining a good sense of humor, learning how to work effectively with a variety of different patient and medical staff personalities, spending time with friends and family, and having interests outside of medicine. I will bring to my residency energy, enthusiasm, a strong work ethic, and a constant desire to learn new things and share ideas with others. I am seeking a challenging, engaging environment in which to learn and deliver high quality care to patients. I hope to help myself and others fully develop our talents so that our patients can achieve optimal health, mobility, and function. I am looking forward to a challenging career in orthopedic surgery involving patient care, teaching, and future discovery.

---

[12]Reproduced, with permission, from the Medschool.com Community website (http://students.medschool.com).

# Personal Statement Samples: Otolaryngology[13]

*I have always been driven by meeting new challenges, and it is that aspect of otolaryngology that is most attractive to me. The spectrum of ENT, ranging from microsurgical procedures of the ear to large head and neck cancer surgery, is one enjoyed by few medical specialties. ENT also encompasses allergy, infectious disease, and endocrinology to name a few areas, and it is this broad scope of possibilities that has drawn me to the field. I am excited about working in a surgical specialty that gives me the opportunity to provide both primary and specialized care to patients of all ages.*

*I gained exposure to ENT during a surgical elective that was part of my third year surgery clerkship. I had just completed my internal medicine rotation and was considering a career in medicine when I was introduced to otolaryngology. The ENT physicians I had the pleasure of working with demonstrated great knowledge of general medicine combined with excellent surgical skills. They had very good rapport with their patients, and they appeared to be some of the most satisfied physicians I have seen in my years as a medical student. They gave me hands-on experience both in the clinic and the operating room. By the end of my surgery rotation, I knew that I would be happiest pursuing ENT as my specialty.*

*I have worked hard during medical school to put myself in a position to be competitive for residency training in the specialty of my choice. I believe my work ethic stems from being raised on a dry land cotton farm in West Texas. I was taught that people are judged by their integrity and their hard work, and any effort I made was expected to be the best I could muster. These values have served me well in all aspects of my life. They have provided me academic success at all levels, and they have been reflected in my clinical evaluations in each rotation. I also believe that my success in medical school is due in large part to my balance between my family and school. I am married to a terrific woman who has encouraged me at each turn, and I have a wonderful four-year-old daughter who keeps my world and priorities in perspective.*

*Outside of school and family, I enjoy golfing, hunting, fishing, and exercising. I have recently taken an interest in photography, and I plan to concentrate this hobby on wildlife and nature photography. My wife and I are expecting our second child, and we are all eagerly anticipating the arrival of the next addition to our family. This is an exciting, changing time in our lives, made all the more so by the prospect of a career in otolaryngology.*

---

[13]Reproduced, with permission, from the Medschool.com Community website (http://students.medschool.com).

*"To Dr. Karen, with love, Timmy and family."* This was the inscription on the inside cover of an 1899 edition of *The Merck Manual* that Timmy's mom gave me on the last day of my pediatrics rotation. At the bottom of the page, in royal blue marker, was the scribbled signature of a three-and-a-half year old, *"Tim."*

Timmy had mitochondrial encephalomyopathy. The clinical picture of his illness early on was that of failure to thrive, and he continued to have waxing and waning episodes of muscle weakness and neurological deficits, including a significant degree of hearing loss. He taught me to sign "lion" and "tiger" because these were two of his favorite stuffed animals; the reason he taught me to sign "see ya' later alligator" is self-evident. He and his family struggled through several misdiagnoses, including cerebral palsy, until the presence of "ragged red fibers" on a muscle biopsy led to the correct diagnosis. I remember wondering at the time what ragged red fibers looked like under the microscope, and wishing that I could see them myself.

Then there was Chase. He was six months old, an ex-23-week preemie, third of triplets. He had spent all but four days of his life in the hospital, suffering from multiple complications stemming from his birth history and necrotizing enterocolitis in his perinatal period. His last night was also my last on call during my pediatrics rotation. I wept after watching my attending stand stoically with his hand on the shoulder of Chase's mother as she held her dying boy. The next day, after just 15 minutes of sleep, I was working in a primary care clinic that was about 25 miles away. I drove 70 miles-an-hour back to the hospital after receiving a call that the pathologist wanted me to attend the autopsy. Nothing unexpected was found on the gross, but I was strangely excited a few days later when the pathologist showed me the micro, which revealed gut bacteria in nearly every organ system.

Before entering medical school, I decided to be a pediatrician. As pathology continued to intrigue me during clinical rotations, I faced a dilemma. Pathology was exciting, interesting and fun, but the lack of patient contact gave me serious doubts. Would I feel like less of a doctor if I never met another Timmy or held another Chase? I was born to blue-collar parents, grew up in a blue-collar neighborhood in Chicago, and had blue-collar friends. I wanted to make my parents—especially my father—feel proud. My mom trained my nephew to say "Auntie Doctor" any time he saw a woman with a stethoscope. Friends pledged to bring their sick children to me someday. Would they all be less proud of me if I never wrote a prescription, never again used my stethoscope, if they couldn't see that I too would help heal people because they didn't understand what I did?

So I delayed the decision. I started my fourth year still answering "I'm not sure," to questions about my specialty choice. Then I began a pathology elective and sought the advice of my attendings. They were offended when I asked questions like, "Were you ever disappointed that you won't ever make anyone better?" They reminded me that their work makes a difference every time one of them calls the results of a frozen section back to the OR, or determines whether a lesion was merely dysplasia or carcinoma in situ, or looks at a bone-marrow to see if chemotherapy has been effective. I was ashamed at having asked the question.

It is possible that no one will ever again call me "Dr. Karen." It is probable that I will never again receive a gift from a patient. And I am not holding my breath for Christmas cards. But I will make patients better. I will make a difference in their lives by giving them the peace of mind of knowing what caused their loved one's death, or perhaps by finding what everyone else missed to provide a diagnosis. I will be excited and challenged and I will have fun as a pathologist. Whether or not my dad will ever understand what ragged red fibers are, remains to be seen.

---

[14]Reproduced, with permission, from the Medschool.com Community website (http://students.medschool.com).

When I was in kindergarten and got asked the question "What do you want to be when you grow up?" There were really only two acceptable answers. I could either choose a life of fighting crime as a policeman or extinguishing blazing infernos as a fireman. I chose fireman. As I got older the same question became more difficult to answer because the choices become more varied and the decision held more gravity. The question wasn't so simple to answer anymore. I went through third year rotations in a quandary about this decision when it suddenly became so simple. I want to do something where I wake up in the morning and can't wait to get to work, and at the end of the day I am sad to leave. This is pediatrics for me. Some say that children are just little half-sized adults but I choose to differ. They are their own individuals. Children possess an honesty about them that adults have lost somewhere along the way and they will openly share with you this honesty about them that adults have lost somewhere along the way and they will openly share with you this honesty. I still remember Maria, the 2-year-old with acute gastroenteritis that hugged me and planted on my cheek the biggest, wettest kiss I have ever had the pleasure to receive. She was convinced I was the one that made her feel better. Of course there was also Mikey, a 4-year-old with a sprained wrist who was very verbally profound in how much distaste he had towards me after I attempted to manipulate the wounded wrist. Then there are the difficult cases that eternally remain etched in your brain. Karen, an 8-year-old with eczema herpeticum that had spread to cover both eyes and eventually sealed both her eyes shut. It is experiences like these that can cause a person to hesitantly leave the floor at the end of a hectic day and want to come back in morning hopeful to see what a new day has in store.

Several other experiences also shaped my decision to enter into pediatrics and work with children. During my undergraduate years at a large public university I was involved in a study of methylphenidate in children with attention deficit disorder. Being a psychology major I found the research extremely intriguing and found myself enjoying spending time with the "difficult" children. While in medical school I worked with the Department of Child and Adolescent Psychiatry at Westchester Medical Center developing an alternative method of therapy for reaching children and adolescents diagnosed with both a history of substance abuse and physical abuse. This was based on previous studies, which demonstrated that traditional "talk" therapies are not as effective for children who have suffered severe emotional distress. For these types of patients other modalities of creative expression had to be developed. This proved to be one of the most challenging and equally rewarding projects I ever had the opportunity to be involved in.

For my current project I have chosen to take a different venue in childcare. I am currently in the process of compiling the research for my master's thesis in public health. I chose to pursue a joint MD/MPH degree after being inspired by other physicians with MPH degrees that I worked with at the National Institutes of Health. My thesis centers on the topic of pediatric emergency room utilization in a metropolitan area. I hope to provide evidence of incorrect utilization of the emergency room for nonemergent health issues and under utilization of the primary care physician for these nonemergent situations. In addition, I will attempt to establish that incorrect utilization of the emergency room may have indirectly contributed to the rising cost of healthcare. In the future, I plan to use my MPH as tool to create positive changes not only in ER pediatrics but also in the field of pediatrics in general. Whether it is in the area of maternal-child health or even policy for prevention of pediatric disease, I have a goal to be able to make a difference in the realm of child healthcare.

So what do I want to be when I grow up? I want to be challenged every single day of my life. I want to feel the satisfaction that what I do improves the lives of children in big and small ways. Most importantly, I want to be enamored by the work I do . . . I want to be a pediatrician.

"A very good one!" That's the way I answer people when they ask me what kind of doctor I am going to be. This has been my answer since I started medical school. Growing up in a family of six, with two educators as parents, I was taught to strive for excellence in whatever I do. Although the start of my medical career was somewhat turbulent, over the last two years I have demonstrated this attribute in all of my medical school activities. I must say that taking a leave of absence from my medical education was one of the best things I could have done. It enabled me to refocus my life and rededicate myself to medicine. Never has my determination to become a physician been stronger.

I have chosen to pursue a career in Physical Medicine and Rehabilitation for three main reasons. First, I am intrigued by the area of study. Throughout my medical education, I have been very interested in neuro-muscular medicine. I can remember back to anatomy lab when I was amazed at the way our neurological system was "wired" to the rest of our bodies. Never during my basic science education was I more curious; an elective rotation in PM&R solidified this interest even more. I look forward to the challenges of treating patients in this field.

The multidisciplinary approach to patient care is another reason I like PM&R. I have always felt that the team approach to almost anything was the best way to go about things. I see myself as a "team player." My interpersonal skills are very good and my abilities to lead a group have been demonstrated as the director of a summer camp. Sitting in on "team rounds," I found a great sense of accomplishment in seeing that all of these people were working towards a common cause. I can see how the ultimate goal of helping the patient is better met in this setting.

The last reason I have chosen PM&R as a specialty is my appreciation of the way that this field approaches the patient. I have always felt that patients should be seen as individuals, not cases. I have found that PM&R, unlike most other fields, pays very close attention to the psychosocial aspects of medicine. Patients are seen as mothers, husbands, students, and workers, etc. I feel that this is the only way to truly deal with the care of patients. It is relatively easy to "treat" a disease, but only through a holistic approach can one hope to "heal" a patient.

As a candidate for residencies, I feel that I possess traits that many programs are seeking: Enthusiasm, a strong work ethic, and a positive attitude. I have often been told that the vigor with which I approach life is contagious, and that my upbeat attitude is appreciated by many of the patients I have seen. I work hard at whatever I am doing, yet have the ability to put life into perspective. I believe that these aspects of my personality will make me an asset to any residency program.

In summary, I am an enthusiastic, hard working individual with a positive attitude who is dedicated to the field of Physical Medicine and Rehabilitation. I hope that I will be given the chance to elaborate these thoughts in an interview with your program.

---

[16]Reproduced, with permission, from the Medschool.com Community website (http://students.medschool.com).

# Personal Statement Samples: Psychiatry[17]

*The story is told of the late Wilfred Bion that another analyst once consulted with him regarding the case of a schizophrenic who would wake up in the middle of the night to see if he was really there. Bion thought for a moment and then commented, "Well, everyone deserves a second opinion." Indeed, when I informed my family and friends of my choice to go into psychiatry, I found myself with more "second opinions" than I had ever bargained for. One resident told me he was surprised, since he thought I was very motivated and interested in medicine. Other medical students commented enthusiastically that they admired me for choosing such a difficult field. Invariably, this was followed by a story about a person they had heard about who had left surgery—or obstetrics, or medicine—to become a psychiatry resident, after a psychotic episode in which he or she had almost killed several patients. Strangely enough, no one could tell me which program the resident was in.*

*My interest in psychiatry comes from several different perspectives, which is probably why I find the various biological, social, and psychodynamic aspects of psychiatry so interesting. As a psychology major at Princeton, my courses were mainly biologically and pharmacologically oriented. I wrote my sophomore and junior papers on the psychobiology of seasonal affective disorder (SAD), and then spent two summers in Oxford studying the epidemiology of SAD. Yet, driven by a deeper desire to be able to understand and communicate with as many people as I could, I also studied three different languages at Princeton, was a peer counselor, and sang with three choruses concurrently. After college, I taught mentally retarded and emotionally disturbed adolescents, where I learned how to talk to and work with children who had problems ranging from autism to severe hyperactivity, and also spent much of my free time in the deaf community, where I learned about cultural values and the responses to societal pressures in closed communities.*

*Upon my arrival at medical school, I didn't know if I would go into psychiatry. I was fascinated with how the human body worked, and thought that the cerebral challenge of diagnosing physical disease might be more compelling than the gentle and creative exploration toward understanding the origins of a woman's depression or personality disorder. However, my unconscious betrayed me—I spent much of the time with my medical inpatients talking about what their illnesses meant to them or how their families dealt with their hospitalization. Throughout my third year, I found myself sitting with patients like the young woman at the OB/GYN clinic who admitted with shame that she was being hit by her boyfriend; a gigantic nightclub bouncer at the ambulatory clinic complaining of fatigue, who was just starting to adjust to regular life again after being in jail for 11 years; and a middle-aged woman with unexplained chest pain in the ICU, who cried and held my hand as she told me about months of insomnia and sadness following her painful divorce. I knew this was what I wanted to do.*

*As for the future, I still love research and will be doing a few months of research this year on the topic of memory in survivors of childhood trauma, but I also have a strong leaning toward psychotherapy and am giving serious consideration to becoming trained as a psychoanalyst. Eventually, I would like to have a career in an academic setting, where I can focus on patient care using both psychodynamic and psychopharmacologic techniques, and also teach and do some writing or research. Yet, wherever my future lies in these changing times, I know that as long as I have the unique opportunity and privilege to sit with people, listen to them, and help them tell their stories, I will always be satisfied.*

[17]Reproduced, with permission, from the Medschool.com Community website (http://students.medschool.com).

# Personal Statement Samples: Radiation Oncology[18]

*My decision to become a physician was influenced by several factors that led me to pursue a career in an oncologic subspecialty. My grandmother was diagnosed with breast cancer that later metastasized. My grandfather was diagnosed with lung cancer after having smoked for over thirty years. Recently, my cousin was diagnosed with melanoma, which later spread throughout his body. He was treated with advanced oncologic treatment, including radiation therapy, before passing away a few months ago. These experiences, along with a family friend who is a Radiation Oncologist, solidified my goals to become a Radiation Oncologist. Helping my family has given me an understanding and sensitivity for treating cancer patients.*

*Before learning about cancer through first hand experience, I worked with cancer patients while volunteering at local hospitals while at the University. Volunteering was invaluable because the patients were very eager to share their experiences with me. I was fascinated in biochemistry classes and research by the interactions of genes, normal and mutated, that lead to neoplastic growth.*

*While working towards my M.D. degree at the State University of Medicine, my interests were again fueled by classes and conferences concerning oncology. I started my third year with a Surgical Oncology rotation under Dr. A.L. and Dr. F.M., who challenged me and taught me the surgical aspects of treatment. Dr. R.E., my preceptor for Gynecologic Oncology, allowed me to participate in Tumor Board conferences. These increased my awareness of the risks and benefits of the numerous gynecologic treatment modalities.*

*Radiation therapy engages my interest because of the chance to cure and offer palliation in a minimally invasive to non-invasive manner. I am gratified to be involved in a treatment modality that offers relatively immediate and anatomically directed results. I am amazed by the wide spectrum of clinical cases one sees as a Radiation Oncologist. I also saw patients treated for heterotrophic bone growth and management of cardiac transplant rejection. Through research, I am involved in two projects at S. Cancer Center with the Radiation Oncology department. One project entails biliary duct carcinoma and the other involves spinal cord carcinomas and gliomas. I am also comfortable offering palliation to terminally ill patients because I know that advances will shift to an increasing improvement in treatment and hopefully cure.*

*I have discovered many things about myself. Clinically, I can easily establish rapport with my patients. My evaluations consistently commend my ability to form strong patient-physician relationships. If I did not know the answer to a patient's question, taking the time to learn from and consult with an attending or resident allows me to answer the patient. There is no greater tool for learning than teaching someone else and in that light I hope to remain in an academic setting as my career progresses. I am a diligent worker and excellent time-manager. I will happily spend extra time with a patient because as Dr. A.W., my preceptor in Radiation Oncology, says, "When I am with you, YOU are my only patient."*

*During my residency I wish to obtain excellent clinical and academic training that will provide a strong foundation for a successful and fulfilling career in both an academic and community setting. A quote I found in a book reminds me of the difference I hope to make in people's lives:*

> *"A hundred years from now it will not matter what my bank account was, the sort of house I lived in, or the car I drove . . . but the world may be different because I was important in the life of a patient."*

---

*Sure I will become a doctor. But what field of medicine will I choose? To find the answer to this ever-present question, I entered my clinical clerkships with an open mind, looking to discover my strengths and interests. As I went through my third year clerkships I saw appeal in each experience, however, as the year came to a close I still had not found a niche. I began to look beyond the core clerkships I took as a third year student. The vast number of career options for aspiring physicians can be quite overwhelming. So I decided to persevere in the manner in which I undertake most tasks. I stood back and thought, evaluating positives and negatives, and evaluating myself. I realized that perhaps the best fit for me was possibly something that I had exposure to during every third year clerkship, yet its intricacies and true definition were still very foreign. This field was radiology.*

*Radiology can easily be taken for granted by an inexperienced medical student such as myself. It is ingrained in our heads that to rule in or rule out certain diagnosis on our differential often requires a visual study. The patient goes off to another place and receives this visual study, and soon thereafter a report is made revealing the medical situation that is occurring beyond the human eye. What this place is like and what the people do there began to capture my interest. It seemed quite ideal for a person such as myself who found interest in each clerkship I was exposed to during my third year. It allowed diagnosis in the medically ill, in the young child and infant, in the psychiatric patient with mental status changes that cannot be ruled out by history and physical alone, and of course, it allowed diagnosis in the surgical candidate. Radiology in a sense allows exposure to the entire potpourri of medical specialties, therefore, allowing continuing diversity but from a specialized viewpoint.*

*Realising the specialty that appeals to you is one step; deciding whether you feel you can succeed and contribute in that area is the second. As an incoming resident I feel I have many attributes that suit me to be successful in radiology. First, I feel that the old adage that all radiologists sit in a dark room away from all other human contacts is incorrect. Interpersonal skills are essential for a successful radiologist. Patient contact does occur, although on a limited basis, and interaction with other physicians, whether as a consult or fellow radiologist occur on a daily basis. I enjoy interacting with others and feel my personal skills will provide a comfortable environment for patients and colleagues. Second, I enjoy variety, but at the same time realize that I prefer to focus within a specialty. I enjoy anatomy and anatomic relationships, which is also applicable in the field of radiology. Third, I have come to learn that I am quite visual in both my approach to learning and in my everyday tasks. The field of radiology allows me to take advantage of this ability. I have also always enjoyed solving mind puzzles and games. Radiology allows me to take these visual puzzles, if you will, and put the pieces together to make a differential.*

*A career in radiology provides the challenges and intellectual interests that I desire in my chosen field of medicine. I feel that not making a career choice until after evaluating every clinical experience with an open mind allows me the assurance that I have made the correct decision. Given the opportunity, I feel I have the abilities and determination to succeed and develop into a competent radiologist. My success throughout medical school helps to demonstrate my drive and self-motivation. I have confidence in my abilities, enjoy working as a member of a team, and feel I can be a strong advocate for my patients. With my skills and motivation I feel I will be a valuable member to the field of radiology.*

---

[19]Reproduced, with permission, from the Medschool.com Community website (http://students.medschool.com).

# Personal Statement Samples: Urology[20]

I performed my first surgery at the age of twelve on a Boy Scout campout. My surgical staff, the other members of Troop 148, watched around the operating/picnic table as my attempts to clean the only fish caught that day developed into an exploration of fish anatomy. I was fascinated by the intricate anatomy of living things. I eventually realized that surgery was not only an exploration but also a chance to heal. During my high school years, my mother was diagnosed with a rare cancer of the kidney. Despite a nephrectomy and short periods of hope, the cancer eventually metastasized to her liver. Surgery was no longer an option for her and she began a difficult path of chemotherapy. She died a few years later, but her death did not dim my surgical aspirations. Rather, it made me determined to become a surgeon who strives to improve surgical treatments while maintaining empathy for the suffering of my patients. My research, teaching, and clinical experiences have strengthened this resolve and have helped me to choose urology as my future career.

My research experience began during my undergraduate education. Intrigued by the challenges and complexities of basic science research, I continued my research endeavors during my first and second years of medical school. I worked with Dr. D.U. investigating the use of antigen cytokine fusion proteins as a means of achieving antigen specific alterations of the immune response. I also participated in clinical research during my final two years of medical school. I worked with Dr. P.E. on a retrospective study to evaluate the utility of preoperative CT scan in staging patients with colon cancer. I enjoyed the intellectual challenge of laboratory and clinical research and realized its potential to improve patient care. The field of urology is rich in research opportunities and I look forward to continued involvement in research both in residency and beyond.

I was given unique teaching opportunities in medical school, being selected as a teaching assistant for human anatomy and as a USMLE review course instructor. As an anatomy teaching assistant, I led daily small group discussions and cadaveric dissections. I gained a deeper appreciation of the complexity and variability of the human body while increasing my communication and teaching skills. I enjoy teaching and helping my peers to learn. I look forward to the opportunity to both teach and learn from my patients and colleagues as an academic urologist.

My clinical rotations were especially influential in my decision to become an urologist. I enjoyed all of my clinical rotations and hoped to find a surgical specialty that would offer a similar diversity of clinical experiences. To me, urology provides an ideal blend of surgical precision and medical management and a wide spectrum of patients and problems. In the future, I would like to specialize in one of the many available subspecialties in urology. I am especially interested in urologic oncology.

Surgery, whether on a picnic table or in a sterile room, still inspires me as it did as a child. My research, teaching, and clinical experiences in medical school have been instrumental in focusing that interest to the surgical specialty of urology. My knowledge has grown since my first fish surgery, but I still feel the awe at the complexity of anatomy and how much more there is to learn. I look forward to the ongoing opportunities to learn and contribute as I strive to advance treatment and patient care within the field of urology.

---

[20]Reproduced, with permission, from the Medschool.com Community website (http://students.medschool.com).

# Gearing Up for Interviews

You can breathe a small sigh of relief when invitations for interviews start coming in. You have cleared the first major hurdle in the match process, and your foot is in the door of several programs at least. Now, how to maneuver the rest of yourself through the doorway.

## HOW DO I PREPARE FOR THE INTERVIEW?

Good preparation for program interviews is essential to making the best impression. Being overtired, disorganized, inappropriately dressed, or upset about travel glitches can only hurt. In this chapter we will walk you through the stages of interview preparation.

### Scheduling Interviews

Many program directors will tell you that the date of your interview should not make a difference; however, conventional wisdom favors choosing the latter half of the interview season, so that committee members will better recall your application during the ranking sessions. For many applicants, the crucial period is after Christmas.

As a result, during the peak interview months of January and February, last minute scheduling changes are very difficult. In addition, travel to the Northeast is especially unpredictable. The Blizzard of 1999 forced thousands of applicants to cancel or reschedule key interviews. If you are in an early match, you will be interviewing from September through December. Remember, if you want maximal flexibility in interview planning, you **must** turn in your ERAS application or paper applications early.

The interview process can be more grueling than you think. For starters, **don't schedule interviews too close together.** Space them at least 2 days apart so that you'll have time to travel, recuperate and digest information from the previous interview. Schedule the most competitive and desirable programs in the middle of your interview schedule. By then you should reach peak interview form without having lost your enthusiasm and energy (Figure 8–1). In fact, many applicants end up canceling interviews near the end of the season from pure fatigue. If you decide you do not want or cannot make an interview appointment, inform the program as far in advance as you

INTERVIEWS LATER
IN THE SEASON ARE
MORE MEMORABLE BUT
ARE ALSO MORE OF A HASSLE.

SCHEDULE THE MOST
COMPETITIVE AND YOUR
MOST DESIRABLE PROGRAMS
IN THE MIDDLE OF YOUR
INTERVIEW SCHEDULE.

**FIGURE 8-1**

PERIOD OF PEAK PERFORMANCE

INTERVIEW SAVVY

ENTHUSIASM

EARLY    MIDDLE    LATE
INTERVIEW SEASON

Performance during interview season.

can, so that they can fill your interview slot with another applicant. It's simple courtesy. Bear in mind that reports of bad manners travel far in the small circle of residency program directors.

Try to arrange interviews in geographical clusters, so that you can easily drive between sites or take advantage of cheaper regional travel options. (See the section "Planes, Trains, and Automobiles.") It is not inappropriate to politely request an interview at a specific program if you will be traveling to that general area for other interviews. Ask if rounds or a morning conference is a scheduled part of the day's activities. If not, ask if you can attend one or the other. Rounds/conferences are often one of the easiest and most useful ways to judge the style and caliber of a program.

## Mock Interviews

When you hit the interview trail, you will want to be in fine shape. Real interviews are time-consuming and take serious effort to set up. **Never** treat a real interview as a practice session, even if it is at one of your less desirable programs. You never know how a visit will affect your rankings, especially if you end up bumping one of your lower-ranked choices to the top of your "most wanted" list.

After 4 years in school, however, anyone could lose their interviewing finesse. To get a little practice before the real thing, set up a mock interview with your career adviser or another faculty member in the department. Ideally, this person will be an active member of the selection committee in your specialty. Before you go in for your mock interview, review Chapter 9. Have your "interviewer" conduct a "tough" interview with hard questions, especially if he or she has a reputation as a "softy." Otherwise, he or she should treat you like any other candidate who walks through the door. Afterwards, your "interviewer" should give you detailed feedback on your ease/confidence in handling the questions, the quality of your answers, and other personal qualities that you projected during the interview (eg, maturity, thoughtfulness, intelligence, ability to think quickly, etc).

If you want to squeeze even more feedback out of the ersatz interview, you can have it videotaped or audiotaped, and then review it with your "in-

ROUNDS AND CONFERENCES
PROVIDE GLIMPSES
OF THE PROGRAM'S SOUL.

terviewer." Try to evaluate yourself from his or her perspective. You can also simulate other aspects of the interview by coming to the "office" in full interview dress, carrying a folder of materials, and being forced to stew a few minutes outside with the secretary because the interviewer is currently with another applicant. Likewise, you can assemble as complete an application file as possible, have the "interviewer" review it, and ask you questions based on your file. For the truly obsessive-compulsive, there are even professionals who can play the interviewer, videotape the session, and coach you to a fine-tuned performance.

## Doing Your Homework for the Road

A few days before any actual interview, call the institution to confirm the date, time, location, and interviewers. If you have any of their names, build on this knowledge. Is your interviewer a researcher, a clinician, a house officer, or an administrator? Then get to work: (1) Call up local contacts (ie, graduates from your school currently in the program), or ask the program's administrative assistant about the interviewer's specialty, personality, etc.; (2) Run a MEDLINE search (available free through Medschool.com at http://students.medschool.com) on the interviewer(s) and read their abstracts. Try to discover mutual interests to potentially discuss during your interview. For the Internet savvy applicant, use AltaVista (http://www.altavista.com) to run a Web or Usenet search on the interviewer's name. (3) Check out the program's departmental website (if applicable) to learn more about the faculty and program. The goal is not to appear political or "calculated," but to be prepared to highlight any strengths you have that might appeal to the interviewer. Even if what you learn does not come up in conversation, you will gain a psychological advantage just from knowing something about the interviewer. He or she already knows a great deal about you; doing your homework offers you a chance to even the playing field a little. In preparation for the interview, you want to organize the following information about each program (Figure 8–2).

Place all this material in a labeled folder. If you have time, review this material and jot down questions and concerns that come to mind for that program. You should also create a folder of your own application materials (Figure 8–3).

Of course, the residency director will also have this information—plus your application—in front of her when she interviews you, all of which is fair game.

**LEVEL THE INTERVIEW PLAYING FIELD BY LEARNING ABOUT YOUR INTERVIEWERS.**

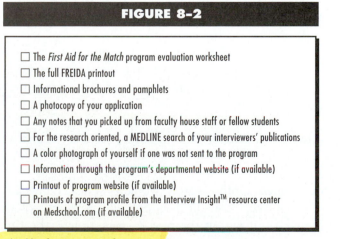

### FIGURE 8-2

☐ The *First Aid for the Match* program evaluation worksheet
☐ The full FREIDA printout
☐ Informational brochures and pamphlets
☐ A photocopy of your application
☐ Any notes that you picked up from faculty house staff or fellow students
☐ For the research oriented, a MEDLINE search of your interviewers' publications
☐ A color photograph of yourself if one was not sent to the program
☐ Information through the program's departmental website (if available)
☐ Printout of program website (if available)
☐ Printouts of program profile from the Interview Insight™ resource center on Medschool.com (if available)

Checklist for program information.

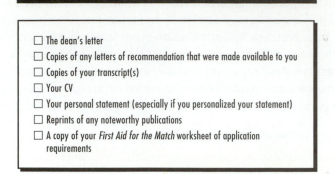

**FIGURE 8-3**

☐ The dean's letter
☐ Copies of any letters of recommendation that were made available to you
☐ Copies of your transcript(s)
☐ Your CV
☐ Your personal statement (especially if you personalized your statement)
☐ Reprints of any noteworthy publications
☐ A copy of your *First Aid for the Match* worksheet of application requirements

Checklist for folder of application materials.

## Interview Attire and Grooming

**General Tips.** Remember, you are trying to get a job as a doctor, so dress like one. Both men and women should dress conservatively but stylishly. Clothing and shoes should be comfortable, since most interviews will include tours of the facility. You might want to bring a small leather briefcase or a neat folder containing blank paper, pen, and extra copies of your CV and personal statement. Since most of the interviews will be conducted in the late fall or winter, dress for warmth, particularly if you are interviewing at programs in the Snowbelt. Always ask another person to inspect your appearance in your interview suit to make sure that you project a professional, polished image. Don't forget to schedule a haircut or trim before you take your show on the road, particularly if your hair loses all shape or style when overdue for a trim. Finally, if you do use fragrance or aftershave lotion, go easy with the dosage. You want to be remembered for your "stylish young doctor" look, not for filling the room or elevator with a thick cloud of fragrance.

**Just for Men.** Don't assume that your suits from your medical school interviewing days still fit. Try them on several months in advance. If they no longer fit or are not in style and cannot be easily altered, consider a shopping trip. If you want custom-tailored suits, get measured for them at least 2 months before your interviews begin. If you buy ready-made suits, tell the salesperson that you are looking for interview suits. If you cannot stand the traditional black, brown and navy, consider olive. In any case, remain with a conservative but classy cut; this is not the time to experiment with avant-garde designer labels. Your shirts should also be conservative in style and color, and made of good-quality material.

Two suits should be adequate for most interview trips. Each suit should be good for two or three interviews. Alternate your suits to let the other suit air out and shed its wrinkles. When there is a break in the interview schedule, you can have the suits dry-cleaned. You might want to pack a portable iron and a lint brush for trips.

Men with fast growing beards: it's not a bad idea to carry a razor so that you can shave right before afternoon interview sessions. A five o'clock shadow can take the edge off your sharp professional image.

**Just for Women.** Unfortunately, women's styles change so quickly that the suits you bought before medical school will probably look dated. Unless you've purchased a suit within the past 2 years, now is the time to splurge

**AVOID LETHAL DOSES OF PERFUME OR AFTERSHAVE.**

and invest in one or two new suits for the interview trips. Although there are many stylish pants suits out there, conservative wisdom prefers the classically cut skirt and jacket ensemble. The jacket must be long-sleeved. The skirt should fall just below, or just above, the knee. When you try the skirt on, march around the dressing room area. If the skirt won't allow you to stride freely, it's wrong for a professional outfit. You'll be doing a lot of walking on your interviews, and you need a skirt that won't hobble you.

AVOID THE "DRUG REP" LOOK.

Although women have more choices than men in suit colors, it's a good idea to stay away from overly bright colors and busy patterns. Similarly, your blouse should be classic in cut, with a neckline that is not too low, and in a color and texture complementary to the suit. Generally, suits made of wool or linen/cotton blends travel best, with the fewest wrinkles and the best fabric weight to adapt to changing weather conditions. Be prepared to spend several days shopping for the right suit. If you have the time, you may want to take your new purchase to a men's tailor for alterations. Unlike men, women are generally not accustomed to having off-the-rack suits altered for a perfect fit, but when 3 or 4 years of your future are at stake, it may well be worth the extra cost. Professional alterations are especially important if you are not a standard size.

CONSIDER PROFESSIONAL ALTERATIONS.

It's difficult to walk the fine line of looking professional and still looking feminine. The shoes that you will be wearing on interview trips should be comfortable, since there may be a lot of walking on slippery hospital floors. Generally, low-heeled pumps in a color complementary to your suits are best, with neutral-colored hosiery. Keep makeup and jewelry to a minimum. Unless you really need one, don't carry a handbag. Instead, opt for a leather attaché case to hold your papers, keys, makeup, and a comb or brush.

## HOW CAN I TRAVEL INEXPENSIVELY?

Unfortunately, interviews will cost most of you a lot of time and money. During the 1999–2000 interview season, for example, students reported spending an average of 20 days away from medical school at their program interviews, and paid $2000 for application fees and travel expenses (Figures 8–4 and 8–5).

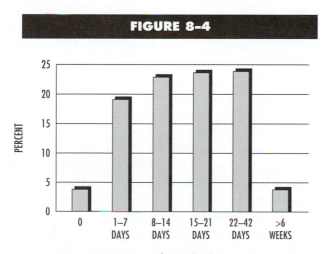

**FIGURE 8-4**

Days spent interviewing away from school.

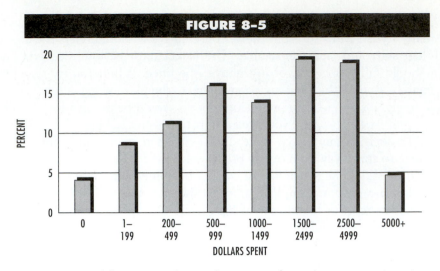

FIGURE 8-5

Amount in U.S. dollars spent applying and interviewing for residency positions (1994).

It's possible in most cases to make travel arrangements for your interviews without razing your bank account. To some extent, the most cost-efficient means of transportation depends on geographical location. Some parts of the United States have better rail service than others. In some areas, a rented car may be your best option. The next section will introduce you to some ways to minimize your travel expenses.

## Planes, Trains, and Automobiles

**American Express Student Services:** If you do not yet have an American Express card with student services, we recommend that you get one. At present, the AMEX student card comes with 4 coupons (2 can be used during the interview season), good for heavily discounted travel on Continental Airlines. If you apply for the AMEX Credit Card for Students instead of the AMEX Card for students, **there is no annual fee.** As this book goes to press, the coupons allow you to purchase a round-trip ticket for $159 if you fly within a zone. There are 3 zones. Zone A is the eastern, southern, and some of the midwestern states. Zone B is the other midwestern states and the western states, except the west coast. Zone C is the west coast states. Round-trip tickets are $219 for travel between cities located in Zone A and Zone B or between cities located in Zone B and Zone C, and $269 for travel between cities located in Zone A and Zone C. The travel dates for the 1999/2000 Amex Student Program were from September 9, 1999 to May 31, 2000. You must make reservations less than 30 days in advance. That means you can make last minute reservations if seats are still available in the appropriate fare class. In addition, you can currently take a companion with you at the same fare. If you are interviewing together as a couple, or if you can coordinate interviews with a friend, you can get extra mileage from the American Express/Continental coupons. Out of coupons? No problem. You can call AMEX for another set of coupons. Be aware of the blackout dates and that there is a minimum stay of one Saturday night. Application processing takes approximately 4 weeks. For further information or to enroll in the Student Services program, call or go to their website:

DON'T LEAVE HOME
WITHOUT IT.

American Express Student Services
(800) 942-2639
http://www.americanexpress.com

**American Airlines Meeting Saver Fares for AAMC Student Residency Interview Program:** Discounts of 5% and 10% on American Airlines fares are available to all medical students during the interview season. The discounts are not enormous; however, you can get them without coupons or membership in any organization. For more information, call:

American Airlines Meeting Services
(800) 433-1790; ask for the new STAR file number for the season
Or you can obtain the STAR file number by e-mailing the AAMC at:
lgordinier@aamc.org

**Discount regional airlines:** Given recent increased competition from low-fare airlines like Southwest, you can obtain very reasonable airfares when traveling regionally (Table 8–1). As with other airlines, tickets are cheapest with a 21-day advance purchase and a Saturday night stay. With discount airlines, you may encounter less choice in flight times and more stopovers.

**Southwest Airlines** (800-IFLYSWA, http://www.iflyswa.com): Southwest has grown rapidly since its inception in 1971 to become the fifth largest airline in the U.S. It takes pride in its low fares and customer service. Their Internet site is extremely user-friendly. After you enter in your travel parameters, the search engine will show you all the available flights along with the corresponding fares listed under the different fare categories. By clicking a few boxes to modify your travel times, you can easily search for the lowest fare available. Southwest services the following cities:

| | | |
|---|---|---|
| Albany | Columbus | Indianapolis |
| Amarillo | Corpus Christi | Islip |
| Austin | Dallas | Jackson |
| Baltimore | Detroit | Jacksonville |
| Birmingham | El Paso | Las Vegas |
| Boise | Fort Lauderdale | Kansas City |
| Burbank | Harlingen | Little Rock |
| Chicago-Midway | Hartford | Los Angeles |
| Cleveland | Houston | Louisville |

**TABLE 8–1. Discount airlines.**

| AIRLINE | REGIONS WITH STRONG COVERAGE | PHONE NUMBER | WEBSITE ADDRESS |
|---|---|---|---|
| Alaska Airlines | West Coast | (800) 426-0333 | http://www.alaskair.com |
| America West | Southwest | (800) 235-9292 | http://www.americawest.com |
| American Trans Air (ATA) | Midwest | (800) I-FLY-ATA | http://www.ata.com |
| Frontier Airlines | Denver, West Coast, and Midwest | (800) 432-1359 | http://www.flyfrontier.com |
| Midway Airlines | Midwest and East Coast | (800) 446-4392 | http://www.midwayair.com |
| Midwest Express | Midwest | (800) 452-2022 | http://www.midwestexpress.com |
| Southwest Airlines | West Coast, Midwest, South | (800) I-FLY-SWA | http://www.iflyswa.com |
| United Shuttle | Both coasts | (800) SHUTTLE | http://www.ual.com |

Source: Roadmap to the Match Resource Center on Medschool.com (http://students.medschool.com).
Contribution: Up to date Match News, links, tips, and student feedback on specific residency programs.

| | | |
|---|---|---|
| Lubbock | Orlando | San Diego |
| Manchester | Phoenix | San Francisco |
| Midland/Odessa | Portland | San Jose |
| Nashville | Providence | Seattle/Tacoma |
| New Orleans | Raleigh/Durham | Spokane |
| Oakland | Reno | St. Louis |
| Oklahoma City | Sacramento | Tampa |
| Omaha | Salt Lake City | Tucson |
| Ontario | San Antonio | Tulsa |
| Orange County | | |

**Low-cost airlines:** These upstart airlines generally provide a price break when compared to the major airlines. They will often not appear in travel agents' computers or on the Internet travel websites, so you probably will need to go to each airline's web page directly.

**Air Tran** (800-247-8726, http://www.airtran.com): Based in Atlanta, it provides service to about 30 cities in the Eastern United States.

Florida: Fort Lauderdale, Fort Myers, Fort Walton Beach, Jacksonville, Miami, Orlando, Tampa
Georgia: Savannah
Illinois/Iowa: Chicago-Midway, Moline/Quad Cities
Indiana: Bloomington
Louisiana: New Orleans
Massachusetts: Boston
Michigan: Flint
Mississippi: Gulfport/Biloxi
New Jersey: Newark
New York: Buffalo/Niagara Falls, New York-LaGuardia
North Carolina: Greensboro/High Point/Winston-Salem, Raleigh-Durham
Ohio: Akron/Canton, Dayton
Pennsylvania: Philadelphia
Texas: Dallas/Fort Worth, Houston-Hobby
Tennessee: Knoxville, Memphis
Virginia: Newport News/Williamsburg
Washington DC: Dulles

**American Trans Air (ATA)** (800-435-9282, http://www.ata.com): Based in Chicago, it has flights to the following cities:

Arizona: Phoenix
California: Los Angeles, San Francisco
Colorado: Denver
Florida: Fort Lauderdale, Fort Myers, Orlando, Sarasota, St. Petersburg
Indiana: Indianapolis
Iowa: Des Moines
Michigan: Grand Rapids, Lansing
Nevada: Las Vegas
New York City: JFK, LaGuardia
Ohio: Dayton
Pennsylvania: Philadelphia

Texas: Dallas
Wisconsin: Madison, Milwaukee

**Frontier Airlines** (800-432-1359, http://www.flyfrontier.com): Based in Denver, it serves:

Albuquerque
Atlanta
Baltimore/Washington
Boston
Bloomington
Chicago-Midway
Dallas/Fort Worth
El Paso
Kansas City
Las Vegas
Los Angeles
Omaha
Orlando
New York-La Guardia
Phoenix
Portland
Salt Lake City
San Diego
San Francisco
Seattle

**National Airlines** (888-757-5387, http://www.nationalairlines.com): Based in Las Vegas, it flies to:

Chicago-Midway
Dallas/Fort Worth
Los Angeles
New York-JFK
Newark
Philadelphia
San Francisco

**Proair** (800-939-9551, http://www.proair.com): Based in Detroit, it serves:

Atlanta
Baltimore/Washington
Chicago-Midway
Fort Myers
Indianapolis
New York-La Guardia
Newark
Orlando
Philadelphia
St. Petersburg

**Spirit Airlines** (800-772-7117, http://www.spiritair.com): Based in Detroit, it provides service to:

Atlantic City
Cleveland
Fort Lauderdale
Fort Myers
Los Angeles
Melbourne
Myrtle Beach
New York-La Guardia
Newark
Orlando
Tampa
West Palm Beach

**Sun Country** (800-752-1218, http://www.suncountry.com): Based in Minneapolis, it provides flights to:

California: Los Angeles, San Diego, San Francisco
Florida: Fort Lauderdale, Fort Myers, Miami, Orlando, Sarasota,
        Tampa/St. Petersburg
Massachusetts: Boston
Michigan: Detroit
Nevada: Las Vegas, Laughlin
New York: JFK
Texas: Dallas/Fort Worth, Harlingen, Houston, San Antonio
Washington, DC: Dulles
Wisconsin: Milwaukee

**Vanguard Airlines** (800-826-4827, http://www.flyvanguard.com): It serves:

Atlanta
Buffalo
Chicago-Midway
Cincinnati
Dallas/Fort Worth
Denver
Kansas City
Minneapolis/St. Paul
Myrtle Beach
Pittsburgh

**Amtrak "All Aboard":** Amtrak's "All Aboard" train travel program allows you three stops within a 45-day period. "All Aboard" divides the country into three geographic regions (Western, Central, Eastern). Fares, which start at $229, increase as you traverse more regions. For more information, call or visit:

Amtrak
(800) USA-RAIL
http://www.amtrak.com

Amtrak also offers a 15% discount off any rail fare to students with a Student Advantage card. There is a $20 annual fee for the card. To apply for the card, visit their website or call (800) 96-AMTRAK

**East Coast light rail:** Because the entire Eastern seaboard is well connected with light rail, rail is a viable alternative to driving, especially given distances of 200 miles or greater. Reasonable fares are available even with little advance reservation or none. To receive general rail schedules for the East Coast, call:

Amtrak
(800) USA-RAIL
http://www.amtrak.com

For the New York metropolitan area and Connecticut, call:

Metro-North
(800) METROINFO
http://www.relonet-intl.com/metronorth.html

In general, rail travel may be a more useful throwback than you think: you can use the time to review interview materials, rest, or catch up on other reading, none of which is possible when you drive.

**Travel agencies:** You can purchase a ticket directly through the airlines described earlier, or you can visit your local travel agency. Student-oriented discount travel agencies include STA Travel (800) 777-0112. Travel agents have access to information about the lowest available airfares on all major airlines. Unfortunately, some discount airlines, like Southwest, are not listed on their computers. Their services are free to you, since their commissions are paid by the airlines. In general, try to purchase tickets 3 weeks in advance for the cheapest fares. Make sure the airport you fly into is the best airport in terms of price and distance from your program destination. You must balance the airfare with the time and cost of a taxi to your lodging.

**Internet travel agencies:** These have proliferated because of their usability and cheap prices. Listed below are some of the more popular sites.

**Priceline** (http://www.priceline.com): This website allows you to name your own price for your airfare. After you enter in your desired travel plans, credit card number, and the amount you wish to pay, Priceline will search for any airline which has an available airfare that matches your criteria. If they find a match, your credit card will be immediately charged. Once purchased, you cannot change, transfer, or cancel your ticket. You should know that although you choose your travel dates, the airline will choose the travel times (which will range between 6 AM and 10 PM). Priceline will search for non-stop flights first, but there is a chance that you will have to make a stop or a connection.

**Cheap Tickets** (http://www.cheaptickets.com): Cheap Tickets has been providing discount airfares on major airlines since 1986. You will need to establish a free profile. Finding fares is easy; the site will lead you through a series of dropboxes. Using your search parameters, the site will then list available flights from which you can form an itinerary. When your search results are shown, you will be told what the lowest available fare is, but you won't be told if a seat is available. You will then need to click on the "Seat Availability" button, but remember that the available seats may not be at the lowest fare. If you did not get a seat at the lowest fare available, click on the "Fare Rules" button to see the restrictions for the lowest fare. You can then try to make modifications to your flight parameters in order to receive the low fare. A Visa, Mastercard, or American Express credit card can be used to purchase flights. Cheap Tickets charges a $7.95 processing fee per order. Be sure to check their "Specials" page, as well as their hotel discount and rental car pages as well.

**Expedia** (http://www.expedia.com): Expedia has a variety of features from which you can check for airfares. You do not need to be a registered member to use the various search engines, but you will have to establish a free member profile if you wish to purchase. Their basic fare search is similar to other websites in that it will search for the lowest airfare once you have typed in your search parameters. Expedia allows you to reserve your flight itinerary until midnight of the following day, but the fare is not guaranteed. Other search options include "Fare Compare," which will list flights similar to yours that other Expedia.com members have found. There is also the "Flight Price Matcher" which employs the same concept as Priceline.com. You get to pick the price you are willing to pay for your flight. If a match is made, your credit card will be charged immediately. Some hints for getting your fare are: (1) travel on a Tuesday, Wednesday, or Saturday, (2) plan a Saturday night stayover, and (3) be flexible about your travel times and connecting flights. As with other sites, Expedia.com has hotel discount and rental car pages.

**Travelocity** (http://www.travelocity.com): Travelocity has the basic airfare, hotel and rental car search engines. It also has a "Fare Watcher" feature, which allows you to pick certain cities that the website will continually look for low fares and post them for you. You will need to register before you can use any of Travelocity's features.

**Preview Travel** (http://www.previewtravel.com): This site features a "9 Best Itineraries/Low Fare Search Engine," which will show the 9 cheapest itineraries based on the customer's parameters. It is a popular website with travelers, and has won many awards for its usability and customer service.

**Lowest Fare** (http://www.lowestfare.com): This site allows you to check airfares and seat availability without having to register first (of course you will have to register to purchase tickets). Be sure to check their specials, which are on their home page. Lowestfare.com also gives you access to maps and weather information in a selected city.

## Where to Stay

You will need to take overnight housing into account as part of your travel plans. It isn't always necessary to figure big bucks into your budget for this item; consider the following possibilities:

**Free or low-cost accommodations arranged by the program:** Some programs, especially primary care programs in the Midwest and East, will provide complimentary or discounted lodging at a nearby hotel or guest house. If your interview situation does not volunteer information about such arrangements, ask the administrative assistant if any are available. Also, you may consider asking the residency program about staying in the residents' call room, if there is one available. Be sure to find out if it will remain unoccupied during the night, so that you will be able to sleep well. Not only will it be free, but you also will not have to worry about finding your way to the hospital on the morning of the interview!

**Housing Extension Network (HEN):** This housing network is a service provided by the Organization of Student Representatives, a section of the AAMC. Any medical school can participate in the network if at least eight medical students at that school are willing to house visiting applicants. Participating hosts need not be fourth-year students. One advantage of arranging housing through HEN, however, is that your host **might** be a fourth-year medical student who can give you the last (or latest) word on the program and the institution. If your school is a HEN participant, a directory of other participating schools and hosts with phone numbers and addresses is available through your student affairs office or class representative. If your school is not a part of HEN, bring the network to the attention of your class officers. For further information call:

AAMC
(202) 828-0682

**For women—AMWA Bed & Breakfast Program:** The American Medical Women's Association has a "Bed and Breakfast Program" for members traveling to residency interviews. A member calls AMWA and specifies her destination. AMWA then supplies her with a list of members in the area, mostly physicians who have agreed to provide short-term (1–3 days) lodging for other members. The student is then responsible for making arrangements with the host. AMWA charges $10 for the referral service; the student pays her host an additional $15. To use the service or for more information, contact:

American Medical Women's Association
801 North Fairfax Street, #400
Alexandria, VA 22314-1767
(703) 838-0500
E-mail: mglanz@amwa-doc.org

**Recent graduates:** Some student affairs offices maintain lists of recent graduates and their residency programs. Not only are recent graduates at your target programs an invaluable source of information about the program, they might offer to put you up for a night when you visit.

**Other applicants:** On the interview trail, you often meet applicants from the schools and institutions that you will later be visiting. They may be friendly enough to offer you housing when you visit their home institution, or just show you around the evening before the interview. If they will also be visiting your school at some point, consider extending them the same courtesies.

**Accommodations recommended by the program:** If you are stumped for housing options or prefer more luxurious surroundings, you can always check out local hotels recommended by the program. Residency programs often make arrangements with a hotel to offer discounts if you mention that you are interviewing with them. This information is often included with written invitations for interviews. If you don't get the official word, you can ask the administrative assistant for suggestions.

**Hostels:** They are cheaper than hotels because you will be sharing living quarters with your fellow travelers. Bathrooms and living rooms are communal, and sleeping quarters usually consist of a dormitory type setting with bunk beds. If you are a light sleeper, consider that you will be sleeping in the same room as other people who may snore or come in late. Hostels are a great idea if you are staying in a city for more than one night, because you will be able to meet others who are interested in exploring the area. Try to find out as much information about the hostel, including the location (is it near noisy nightclubs?) and general atmosphere (party crowd vs quiet folks). Also, ask if travelers are required to complete chores as part of their stay. Hostels are generally safe, but be sure to keep your valuables with you or locked up in the hostel's lockers or safes. Remember that not all hostels take reservations, so have a back-up plan. For more information, check out:

*Hostelling U.S.A., The Official Guide to Hostels in the United States of America.*
Websites: Hostels.com, Hostelling International (www.iyhf.org)

**Lodging Discounts:** Hotel-discount companies that consolidate empty hotel rooms can offer you 20 to 70% off the regular rates if they make your arrangements (Table 8–2). Best availability is usually restricted to the major cities. Don't forget to ask about the cancellation policy before booking. In addition, after getting a rate on a given hotel, check with the hotel directly and find out: (1) its proximity to the residency program; and (2) whether an even lower price is available.

If you know that you'll be doing some significant traveling, consider enrolling in a program that can get you up to a 50% discount off regular hotel rates wherever you travel. The major programs usually include more than 2000 hotels worldwide (Table 8–3). To be eligible for the discount, you usually make a reservation with your membership card number. The discount rate may have limited availability, and sometimes requires a 30-day advance notice. If all goes well, you can end up pampered, save some money and save the highway-motel experience for later.

**Hotel Discounts** (http://www.hoteldiscount.com): This is a very user-friendly site. Simply click on your desired city, enter in your travel dates and number of people, and the site will then provide a list of cheap hotels. You can also get a detailed description of the hotel and a map of the area surrounding the hotel. There is a "Lowest Rate Guarantee" that states: If there is a lower rate found for the same dates and the same hotel, and that rate was available at the time of booking, Hotel Discounts will either refund the difference or cancel the reservations without penalty. Check out their various "Hot deals" and other discounts. If you do not have Internet access, call (800) 715-7666.

**Budget-Priced Chains:** Finally, you can simply go with a budget hotel/motel chain. If the residency program is not helpful with names and numbers of nearby lodging, you can call any of these major chains (Table 8–4). When you make your reservation, ask about the room. Common concerns include a non-smoking room, location in a quiet part of the hotel/motel, and a phone connection. And for security, is there a dead-bolt lock? A peephole in the door?

| TABLE 8–2. Hotel-discount companies. | | |
|---|---|---|
| **Company** | **Number** | **Website** |
| Hotel Reservations Network | (800) 964-6835 | http://www.hoteldiscount.com |
| Quickbook | (800) 789-9887 | http://www.quickbook.com |
| Room Exchange | (800) 846-7000 | N/A |

| TABLE 8–3. Some half-price hotel programs. | | | |
|---|---|---|---|
| Program | Membership Price | Number | Website |
| Encore | $69.95 | (800) 638-0930 | http://www.emitravel.com |
| Entertainment Publications | $24.90 (U.S. hotels ed.) | (800) 445-4137 | http://www.entertainment.com |

**University Dorms.** Many residency programs are located at colleges and universities that rent out empty dormitory rooms for $15 to $30 per night. Unfortunately, programs sometimes neglect to mention such accommodations in their brochures.

## Handy Travel Tips

Lastly, we offer a few additional pointers to make your interview trip as smooth as possible:

1. Plan to arrive at your accommodations no later than the afternoon of the day before your interview. This will give you a chance to get oriented, adjust to time zone differences, and handle any unexpected mishaps (eg, lost luggage). If you are planning to fly out the day of the interview, check with the departmental secretary to make sure that there are no further events scheduled for later that day. About departures: in general, it is better to leave later in the day if possible, so that you can have extra time to talk to house staff and faculty, or to see more of the hospital and facilities.

2. When flying, try to take everything as carry-ons. You can bypass the crowded airport counter for a gate check-in and eliminate the risk of the airline losing your luggage. We suggest a durable garment bag or a

**ARRIVE EARLY; LEAVE LATE**

| TABLE 8–4. Major budget hotel/motel chains. | | |
|---|---|---|
| HOTEL CHAIN | NUMBER | WEBSITE |
| Baymont Inns | (800) 4-BUDGET | http://www.baymontinns.com |
| Clubhouse Inns | (800) CLUB-INN | http://www.wyndham.com |
| Comfort Inns | (800) 4-CHOICE | http://www.comfortinn.com |
| Country Inns and Suites | (800) 456-4000 | http://www.countryinns.com |
| Courtyard Marriott | (800) 321-2211 | http://www.courtyard.com |
| Days Inns | (800) 325-2525 | http://www.daysinn.com |
| Econo Lodge | (800) 4-CHOICE | http://www.hotelchoice.com |
| Fairfield Inn | (800) 228-2800 | http://www.marriotthotels.com |
| Hampton Inn | (800) HAMPTON | http://www.hampton-inn.com |
| HoJo Inn | (800) 654-2000 | http://www.hojo.com |
| Holiday Inn Express | (800) HOLIDAY | http://www.basshotels.com |
| La Quinta | (800) 531-5900 | http://www.laquinta.com |
| Motel 6 | (800) 4-MOTEL6 | http://www.motel6.com |
| Ramada Ltd. | (800) 2-RAMADA | http://www.ramada.com |
| Red Roof Inns | (800) THE-ROOF | http://www.redroof.com |
| Rodeway Inns | (800) 4-CHOICE | http://www.rodeway.com |
| Super8 | (800) 800-8000 | http://www.super8.com |
| Travelodge | (800) 255-3050 | http://www.travelodge.com |

roll-aboard suit carrier for your interview clothing. If you must travel heavy, at least pack your interview essentials (eg, program interview materials, application materials, and interview suit) in a carry-on.

3. Pick up an updated discount travel guide. A particularly useful book (it saved one of us, stranded at La Guardia, several hundred dollars on airfare) is *Travel Smarts: Getting the Most for Your Travel Dollar* (Globe Pequot Press) by Teison and Dunnan. This guide, or a similar book by Consumer Reports, will stretch your travel dollar and minimize traveling hassles without sacrificing comfort.

4. If you plan on driving to most of your destinations, get a good U.S. map/road atlas for trip planning. Carry a pocket local map for each city you visit, or tear out the detail pages from an inexpensive road atlas. If you belong to the American Automobile Association (AAA), call or visit your local office once you know your itinerary. Membership privileges usually include free road maps and customized routing advice. It's also worth inquiring about discounts on car rentals and lodging; many AAA clubs offer coupons for these services. And if you should have car problems en route, an AAA card can often save you much more than the cost of the annual membership fee.

    Before you set off, have your car properly winterized and tuned; ask the service station attendant to check your fluids, tire pressure, and replace your windshield wipers if necessary. Be sure to keep your car registration, inspection and insurance papers, and auto club materials in the glove compartment. If you don't already have one for your car, buy a flashlight and batteries—particularly if you will be driving at night.

5. If you have the time, the interview season can be a great way to mix business and pleasure. You can squeeze in some sightseeing if you have more than a day between interviews. You get to unwind between interviews and learn more about the local attractions in the vicinity of the program.

6. Be sure to check local weather conditions in the city where you will be interviewing before you set off. This is especially important if you are traveling to an unfamiliar part of the country, or if you are flying to a region with an exteme climate.

## REFERENCES

Air Tran website (http://www.airtran.com).
America West Airlines website (http://www.americawest.com).
American Express website (http://www.americanexpress.com).
American Medical Women's Association (AMWA) website (http://www.amwa-doc.org)
American Trans Air (ATA) website (http://www.ata.com).
Amtrak website (http://www.amtrak.com).
Baymont Inns website (http://www.baymontinns.com).
Cheap Tickets website (http://www.cheaptickets.com).
Clubhouse Inns website (http://www.wyndham.com).
Comfort Inns website (http://www.comfortinn.com).
Country Inns and Suites website (http://www.countryinns.com).
Courtyard Marriott website (http://www.courtyard.com).
Days Inns website (http://www.daysinn.com).

Econo Lodge website (http://www.hotelchoice.com).

Encore website (http://www.emitravel.com).

Entertainment Publications website (http://www.entertainment.com).

Expedia website (http://www.expedia.com).

Fairfield Inn website (http://www.mariotthotels.com).

Frommer, Arthur, "Upstart Airlines Offer Downscale Fares," *Los Angeles Times*, May 14, 2000.

Frontier Airlines website (http://www.flyfrontier.com).

Holiday Inn website (http://www.basshotels.com).

Hampton Inn website (http://www.hampton-inn.com).

Hostels.com website (http://www.hostels.com).

Hotel Discounts.com Network website (http://www.hoteldiscount.com).

Howard Johnsons Hotels and Inns website (http://www.hojo.com).

La Quinta Inns website (http://www.laquinta.com).

LowestFare.com website (http://www.lowestfare.com).

Medschool.com website (http://www.medschool.com).

Midway Airlines website (http://www.midwayair.com).

Midwest Express website (http://www.midwestexpress.com).

Motel 6 website (http://www.motel6.com).

National Airlines website (http://www.nationalairlines.com).

Preview Travel website (http://www.previewtravel.com).

Priceline.com website (http://www.priceline.com).

Proair website (http://www.proair.com).

Quickbook website (http://www.quickbook.com).

Ramada Ltd. website (http://www.ramada.com).

Red Roof Inns website (http://www.redroof.com).

Rodeway Inns website (http://www.rodeway.com).

Spirit Airlines website (http://www.spiritair.com).

Southwest Airlines website (http://www.iflyswa.com).

Sun Country Airlines website (http://www.suncountry.com).

Super 8 website (http://www.super8.com).

Teison H, Dunnan N: *Travel Smarts*. Old Sanbroot, CT: The Globe Pequot Press, 1995.

Travelocity website (http://www.travelocity.com).

Traveldoge website (http://www.travelodge.com).

United Airlines website (http://www.ual.com).

University of California at San Francisco School of Medicine, *The Next Step: Your Guide to Residency*. San Francisco: University of California at San Francisco, 1995.

Vanguard Airlines website (http://www.flyvanguard.com).

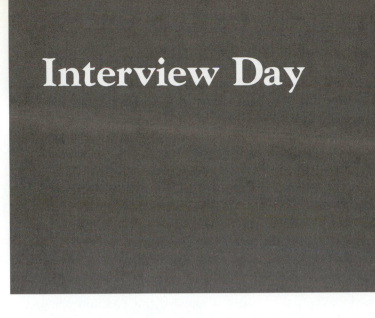

# Interview Day

## WHAT SHOULD I DO THE DAY BEFORE THE INTERVIEW?

By the time you set out on your interview trip, you will want to feel as confident and well prepared as possible. If you have taken our advice in Chapter 8, and planned your arrival for the afternoon before the day of your interview, you will have enough time for these necessary last-minute preparations.

**Review the Program.** Pull out your file on the program you are visiting, including its brochures, your application, the FREIDA printout, etc. Next, review the file of application materials that you had sent to all programs. Try to anticipate interview questions based on your application materials. This step is especially important if your application has some weaknesses. Then make notes on the information you will need to complete your Program Evaluation Worksheet for that program.

**Logistics.** Review your interview itinerary if the program sent you one. Next, orient yourself in the city or town, locate the program offices in relation to your lodging, and make transportation arrangements if you aren't within walking distance of your morning destination. Then, double-check your wardrobe and attaché case; make sure that nothing is missing or damaged.

## TYPICAL EVENTS OF AN INTERVIEW VISIT

No matter what specialty you choose, the visits usually follow the chronology listed below. The interview proper is discussed on pages 135–142. Each segment of the visit represents a different opportunity to learn more about the program, as well as another chance to make a positive impression on the committee members. Be alert; recalibrate your eyes and ears to make the most of each situation, and tailor your questions and responses accordingly. Tune in to your intuition as well; your "gut feelings" may be sending you important warning signals.

## Preinterview Social Events

On the evening before the interview day, programs often invite applicants to dinner with members of the house staff. These meals are typically meant to provide an opportunity for applicants to learn more about the training program in an environment free from the scrutiny of selection committee members. Dress is casual, but avoid jeans and shorts. However, do not be fooled by the relaxed atmosphere; the selection committee usually includes residents and interns. In addition, remember that any strong impression that you leave on any member of the house staff, whether positive or negative, will be communicated to the selection committee.

## Introductions

In the morning of the interview day, you and your fellow applicants will gather in a conference room, where you will (usually) receive a folder containing an itinerary of the day's events, a name tag, a brochure about the training program; and (possibly) call schedules, a summary of benefits, a list of current house officers, and typical house officer rotation schedules. Give the day's schedule priority; read through it carefully, making mental notes of times and places for your interviews. Scan the rest of the packet at your discretion. On interview day itself, pretty color brochures are almost always useless. Save those for later.

After everyone has gathered, you may be addressed by the program director or the chair of the department. It may seem like a routine formality, but give the speaker your full attention. You will usually be able to read the guiding philosophy of the program "between the lines" of the address. As you listen, keep in mind that the preaching and philosophy of the residency director and the department chair heavily shape the program. You will need to ask yourself whether the "shape" of this particular program is compatible with your outlook and goals.

## Tour of Facilities

Most program visits include a tour of the facilities, led by a resident or intern. At programs with multiple training sites, you will usually tour just one hospital in the system, so don't forget to ask questions about the other sites. If there is something you really want to see, your guide will usually be happy to show it to you (Table 9–1). If you can, stay close to your guide; you won't hear anything in the back of the pack. Because your tour leader has to speak so much, you often pick up more unfiltered sentiments and honest opinions than at any other time during your visit.

| TABLE 9-1. Sights to see on a program tour. | | |
|---|---|---|
| **Must See** | **Should See** | **Might See** |
| Wards | Emergency room | Surrounding city |
| ICU | Cafeteria | Fitness facilities |
| Surgical suites | Library/computer resources | Child care facilities |
| Call rooms | | |

**ORIENT YOURSELF IMMEDIATELY TO THE INTERVIEW SCHEDULE.**

## Morning Rounds/Conferences

Every interview itinerary should allow you to see the house staff in action, whether on rounds or in conference. Otherwise, you simply will not get the full picture. Rounds and conferences allow you to gauge the enthusiasm of the house staff, the breadth of knowledge displayed, and the quality of interaction among house officers, staff and faculty. Pay particular attention to the post-call house officers, who tend to be forthcoming in their sleep-deprived state. Your challenge then is to distinguish between grousing due to fatigue and justified grumblings about the program.

## Lunch

Interview lunches range from a meal you buy at the hospital cafeteria to a fancy repast at a downtown restaurant. In any event, eat lightly. If you are stuffed, your concentration and alertness will dissipate as your body focuses on digesting your heavy meal. As with dinner the night before, use lunch as an opportunity to learn more about the program from house staff eating with you and about other programs from your fellow applicants. Avoid messy foods (eg, pasta) that can leave its calling card on your new professional outfit. Because it is tough to maintain a high energy level all day, you might want a cup of coffee or a caffeinated drink to keep you from fading in the afternoon, especially if you have another interview scheduled.

**FEAST ON INFORMATION, NOT FOOD.**

## INTERVIEWING SAVOIR-FAIRE

The interview sessions themselves are usually perceived as the most stressful portion of the interview day. Study after study indicates that these encounters are one of the most important factors in the selection of house staff. Unfortunately, most of these same studies show interviews to have poor predictive value of your future performance as a resident, and show abysmally low reproducibility between interviewers. The bottom line is that the conclusions drawn by an interviewer can often be inaccurate and imprecise. No matter how stellar you are, if the interviewer got up on the wrong side of the bed, you may get toasted anyway. Fortunately for you, interviewers' bad hair days don't happen very often, and most interviews conducted today are low-stress, non-confrontational meetings with a single interviewer. In addition, there are a few things you can do to give yourself the best chance of pulling off a successful interview.

**CONCLUSIONS DRAWN BY AN INTERVIEWER CAN BE INACCURATE.**

Before the actual interviews, learn the pronunciation of your interviewer's name from the departmental secretary or the interviewer's administrative assistant. Arrive at your interviews a few minutes early. If the waiting room makes you anxious, try different relaxation techniques such as deep, steady breathing or alternately tensing and relaxing different muscle groups. It may help your nervousness to remember that interviews often run behind schedule and that experienced interviewers are aware of this tendency. If you are running late, your subsequent interviewer will understand when you explain that your previous interview just finished. When you meet your interviewer, introduce yourself and offer a firm, confident handshake. After being invited into the office, do not sit down until the interviewer sits or invites you to sit.

**DOUBLE-CHECK THE PRONUNCIATION OF YOUR INTERVIEWER'S NAME.**

During the interview, maintain fairly constant eye contact with the interviewer. Do not let your gaze or attention wander, especially when the interviewer is speaking directly to you. Do **not** take notes during the interview; write them down later. Try to project a high energy level, even if this is your fifteenth interview. Answer the questions fully yet avoid rambling; if they want to know more about a particular subject, they will ask. If you can, gently steer the interview toward your strong points, but do not pressure the interviewer or dominate the dialogue; leave filibusters to the politicians. Monitor any signs of nervousness, including fidgeting and pressured speech. **Never** peek at your watch, even if you know that the interview is running overtime. When the interview is finished, thank the interviewer, shake hands again and leave gracefully. Make an effort not to fumble with your folder, purse or briefcase as you rise from your chair.

## WHAT ARE INTERVIEWERS LOOKING FOR?

No matter what specialty interests you, interviewers often seek the same set of qualities in would-be residents. These include character traits in addition to intellectual abilities.

▶ **Intelligence/knowledge.** Does the applicant demonstrate a rich fund of medical knowledge when discussing cases? Is he or she conversant with the history as well as the current issues and challenges defining the specialty?

▶ **Enthusiasm/charisma.** Residency directors consider this to be an invaluable commodity, essential to surviving a long, and often demanding residency. Does the applicant demonstrate liveliness and vivacity? Does he or she appear to have stamina and endurance as well?

▶ **Maturity/insight:** Does the applicant have realistic and appropriate goals? Are his or her responses measured and well-conceived? Can the applicant appraise himself or herself honestly, addressing both strengths and weaknesses?

▶ **Shared philosophy/personality:** Will I enjoy working with this applicant on a regular basis? What do I think this individual will add to this program?

## WHAT DO INTERVIEWERS ASK?

We have compiled a list of the most common interview questions, with suggested approaches for responding.

### Tell Me About Yourself.

A favorite opener. You can respond by asking whether there is anything specific that they would like to know about you, or whether they would like to hear first about your personal or professional background. Otherwise, a short biographical statement will suffice. Because you are asked to summarize your life on this planet in one breath, program directors expect a sense for what you hold most essential. Highlight any unusual or noteworthy interests or experiences, but again, keep it brief. Two additional pointers may be helpful in answering this question: (1) Stress only positive features; (2) Back up generalities with specific illustrations or examples (eg, if you tell the interviewer that you're "research-oriented," briefly describe 1 or 2 of your projects or publications).

## What Are Your Strengths and Weaknesses?

One of the most familiar "tough" questions that surface in interviews. Be ready to summarize your strong points and achievements in three or four concise sentences. The interviewer wants to know whether you can assess your own strengths and weaknesses accurately, and whether you can take appropriate steps to address any deficiencies in your training. The trick is to mention only the deficiencies that tend to be common among your colleagues (eg, weaknesses in ambulatory orthopedics, if you are going into family practice). Do **not** use the worn "my weakness is my strength" ploy. The interviewer will only roll his or her eyes when you "confess" that you are such a perfectionist that you are often unable to leave the hospital before midnight.

## Why Are You Interested in Our Program?

**Why do you want to come here?** Here all your background research and reading pays off. House staff and applicants you meet on the interview circuit can readily identify the strengths and the unique features of the program for you. Stress the philosophies and goals that you have in common with the program, whether dedication to care of the indigent or to high-tech research. If you don't read up on the program before you interview, then you deserve to get burned.

## What Are You Looking for in a Program?

If you have been actively engaged in your application process, then you should be able to answer this question off the top of your head. The interviewer is primarily assessing whether his or her program can meet **your** needs. Highlight the strengths and unique features that make the program attractive to you; do **not** dwell on the program's lackluster areas.

## Why Should We Choose You?

**What can you contribute to our program?** This is almost the reverse of the previous question. To answer this question, you need to reconcile your understanding of the program with a good sense of your own strengths and goals. For example, if the program has an inner-city setting with a large Hispanic population, mention your long-standing interest in indigent health care and fluency in Spanish.

## Can You Tell Me About This Deficiency on Your Record?

The experienced interviewer will be on the lookout for evasions or excuses from applicants who cannot take responsibility for their actions. Be honest and drop the excuses. Be prepared to "take the rap" for any weaknesses in your application. By all means, let the interviewer know if the problem was connected to an unforeseen or unavoidable personal crisis (eg, major illness, divorce, death of a family member). Otherwise, acknowledge the deficiency and offer evidence that you have made a sincere effort to overcome it. If you handle this question well, you will have demonstrated to the interviewer that, while not the perfect applicant (no one is), you have the ability to learn and grow. On the other hand, don't volunteer negative information. Unless you have good reason to believe that something from your past will sink your application, it's poor form to discuss deficiencies not raised by the interviewer.

STRESS PHILOSOPHIES AND GOALS ALSO SHARED BY THE PROGRAM.

## Why Are You Interested in This Specialty?

**What other specialties did you consider and why?** The interviewer wants to verify that your reasons for entering this specialty are both reasonable and genuine. You probably know exactly why you chose one specialty over others; however, it is difficult to verbalize your reasoning on a moment's notice. It helps to formulate a brief answer to this question on paper beforehand. A few words of caution: (1) Lifestyle or monetary prospects are generally considered shallow reasons for entering a particular specialty, so be careful about mentioning these considerations; (2) Do not criticize or put down other specialties in the course of explaining your interest in this specialty. You want to convey the impression that you are attracted to the specialty for its positive attributes, not because you were turned off by everything else.

## What Do You See Yourself Doing in the Future?

Nobody expects you to know exactly what you want to do after your residency, but interviewers do want evidence that you have considered and planned for the most likely career possibilities. Be ready to explore your motivations for these options.

## How Do You Think the Current Changes in Health Care Will Affect the Specialty?

Hopefully, you already asked yourself—and answered—this question when you selected your specialty. If not, you can pick up the current thinking by talking to faculty and house staff in the field or following the specialty journal. Recent changes in health care are unprecedented; and a lot of people are understandably concerned about the long-term implications. Your interviewer will certainly appreciate a well-considered analysis.

## Do You Have Any Plans for a Family?

This is an illegal question that constantly crops up in interviews, especially for female applicants. The interview itself is not, however, the time to lecture the interviewer on the finer points of discrimination in hiring. Answer the question honestly if possible. Otherwise, you can handle it by saying simply, "I have no plans for a family at this time."

## What Do You Do in Your Spare Time?

The interviewer wants to see if you have a life outside of medicine. This is an opportunity for you to allow your personality to shine through. But—try not to sound more enthusiastic about what you do with your free time than about your commitment to medicine!

## Describe an Interesting Case That You Had.

This is a more frequent test of your clinical acumen and your presentation skills. In essence, you are being asked to make a bullet presentation. If this question comes up, begin with a 30-second outline of a case you know well. This should be fully rehearsed but spoken with spontaneity. Lay out the interesting diagnostic or treatment issues facing the team at the time. At this point, the interviewer may join you in a discussion of these issues.

## Other Commonly Asked Interview Questions

Depending on the specialty in which you are applying, there are a handful of other commonly asked interview questions that are more indicative of your

LIFESTYLE AND MONEY ARE GENERALLY CONSIDERED SHALLOW REASONS FOR ENTERING A SPECIALTY.

HOT TOPICS INCLUDE MANAGED CARE, SUPPLY OF SPECIALISTS VERSUS GENERALISTS, AND MEDICARE/MEDICAID REFORM.

interest in a specific specialty. A list of these commonly asked interview questions broken down by specialty are listed in the Appendix of this book. We encourage you to be prepared to encounter questions like these as you go the interview trail.

## WHAT DO I ASK THE INTERVIEWER?

Toward the middle or the end of the session, your interviewer will invariably ask you, "Do you have any questions?" Be prepared in advance with at least two to three questions to show your curiosity and interest, as long as it's appropriate for the interviewer or program. Faculty members can field the more philosophical and broad-based questions like the ones listed below.

An ideal question is one that the interviewer will enjoy answering thus leaving an overall positive tone to the encounter. Remember, however, that you are still the person under observation and evaluation. Do **not** harp on the program's weaknesses. Also, avoid asking questions during the interview about salaries and benefits, vacation, moonlighting, call schedules, and other aspects of the day-to-day operations of the program. Save these practical concerns for the house staff. Keep your interview questions friendly and benign.

### Appropriate Questions for Faculty Interviewers

1. What do you like most about your training program? In what areas can the program improve itself?
2. Where have your residents gone after graduation?
3. What process do you have for improving the residency? For evaluating rotations?
4. Have you ever done "post-marketing" surveys of your graduates? What do they tell you?
5. What recent changes has the program undergone? What changes do you foresee?
6. How many clinicians are there in the program? Researchers/academicians?
7. What research opportunities are available? What is the availability of funding for research? What kind of mentor support is available from the faculty?
8. In what direction do you see the chairperson (or residency director) taking the program? Do you believe that he or she will remain here during my residency training?
9. If there is an interim chair: What is the status of the search process? What changes do you foresee in the program as a result of this transition?
10. What other residency programs do you like and recommend? Why?
11. What opportunities are there to attend regional and national conferences and seminars?
12. How well do the residents perform on board certification exams?
13. What is the structure of the last years of residency? Does the program offer elective time? Mini-fellowships? Time and opportunity to work abroad?

## WHAT TYPES OF QUESTIONS SHOULD I ASK THE HOUSE STAFF?

We compiled a list of questions that you might ask house staff while you are visiting the program. Most of them deal with the daily operation of the resi-

THE QUESTIONS YOU ASK CAN BE REVEALING TO THE INTERVIEWER.

NEVER GRILL THE INTERVIEWER.

dency. A few, however, are sensitive questions that you might not feel comfortable asking all house staff that you encounter (eg, chief residents steeped in the program's "party line"). The sample questions are organized largely by issues discussed in "What should I be looking for in a program?" (p. 61).

## General Questions

1. Are the residents happy? What features of the program do they like or dislike?
2. Would the residents choose the same program again?
3. Does the program have trouble filling all its spots?
4. How strong are the residents? From where did they graduate?

## Location

1. Is the program located in a safe part of the city? If not, what's the security system like?
2. What do residents do for fun around here?
3. What advantages are specific to the location (eg, unusual patient population, cultural opportunities, climate, low cost of living, etc.)?

## Reputation

1. Do graduates of the program have problems finding jobs?
2. How difficult is it for residents to get a good fellowship?

## Education

1. Is the program fully accredited?
2. How are the residents evaluated? By whom?
3. Is there an organized curriculum? What is its emphasis?
4. How many conferences/week are there? Do conferences emphasize practical knowledge or state-of-the-art research?
5. What is the quality of the attendings? What are their responsibilities? Do they get along?
6. How interested are the faculty in the education and welfare of the house staff?
7. What proportion of attendings are private?
8. Are there medical students on the wards? What school(s) do they represent? What are the residents' teaching responsibilities to the students?
9. What research opportunities are there? Are faculty research preceptors readily available?

## Work Environment

1. What is the patient load like?
2. What are the typical admissions diagnoses?
3. How many cases are treated by the average resident?
4. Is the caseload sufficiently varied?
5. How much autonomy do residents have to manage patients?
6. What is the patient population like? Ethnicity/language? Socioeconomic status?
7. Is there continuity of care for patients after discharge?
8. What is the extent and quality of the ambulatory experience?
9. How strong is nursing support? Consult services? Radiology?
10. Pathology? Emergency services?

11. How much "scut work" is done by house staff? Are there blood drawing/IV teams?
12. What is the typical call schedule?
13. How does the work environment vary from service to service? From hospital to hospital?
14. How busy are call nights? How much sleep do you usually get?
15. How available are the attendings? Can you call them at night?
16. Is there backup available when you're on call? Is there a nightfloat system?
17. How many hours do you work each week?
18. How much time do you get off each week?

## Salary

1. What is the starting salary for an intern? For an R2?
2. What about cost of living in the area?
3. Is moonlighting permitted? If so, how does it work around here?

## Benefits

1. What health benefits are available (eg, medical insurance, dental plan, eye plan)?
2. What is the maternity/paternity leave policy?
3. Is life insurance available? Disability insurance?
4. Is parking provided? Is subsidized housing available? What is the vacation schedule setup?

## HOW TO KILL AN INTERVIEW

Given all the time, expense, and adrenaline that contribute to your program interviews, you don't want to blow your chances with an ill-considered question or comment. Therefore, we have provided a checklist of problems that can cost you the interview.

1. **Rambling:** Interviewers probably hear enough poorly constructed medical student presentations as it is. If rambling is just another nervous habit for you, then it should evaporate as you gain experience and become more comfortable with the interview process. If this is not the case, make a more conscious effort to provide complete yet focused answers. You may find that practice sessions with a friendly classmate will help you overcome this tendency.

2. **Not listening/not "reading" the interviewer correctly:** It is easy to fade away briefly during an interview, especially after lunch. However, these TIAs can become big problems if you misunderstand a question that you weren't expecting, or if as a result you ask a question about a topic previously discussed by the interviewer. Most "misreads" can be prevented by simply keeping your attention focused. Use verbal and nonverbal clues to tailor your responses (eg, if the interviewer is a businesslike, impersonal type, don't give "touchy-feely" answers).

3. **Inadequate preparation:** Nobody will expect you to know their program through and through, but you should know its basics. Interviewers do not want to waste the time allotted for the interview going over information already available in their printed materials.

**TAILOR YOUR RESPONSE TO THE INTERVIEWER.**

4. **Grilling the interviewer:** It's true in a philosophical sense that you are interviewing the program as much as they are interviewing you. But be practical: don't put the interviewer on the defensive by harping on the program's weaknesses. If these problem spots are of paramount importance to you, save your concerns for the house staff or raise the issue in a friendly, non-confrontational manner. Interviewers may already be well aware of the weakness, and will be more willing to discuss it if they aren't being made to feel as if they owe you an apology.

5. **Inconsistent/evasive answers:** Answers that don't match up with what you wrote on your application, or that are incomplete will put most interviewers on "red alert." Do emphasize your strengths as well as the clinical and academic interests that you share with the interviewer. Do not exaggerate, lie, or otherwise distort facts. Interviewers expect applicants to be open and honest. Moreover, program directors can and often do verify your claims or credentials by calling colleagues at your school.

6. **Displaying a difficult/quirky personality:** The interviewer is trying to picture you as a junior colleague with whom daily interaction will be necessary. If you come across as domineering, inflexible, temperamental, or eccentric, you will not be making this task a pleasant one.

7. **Pejorative comments about other programs:** Negative statements (especially unsolicited or unsupported digs) about other programs or your own school will be noted as indiscretions that reflect badly on you. The interviewer will wonder what you might say about his or her program at the next place on your tour. The residency community is tight, and the interviewer may very well have colleagues and friends at the programs you just bashed.

8. **Poor interactions with administrative staff/house staff:** It should go without saying that rudeness or lack of consideration for these people will be relayed to the residency selection committee, as a strike against you.

## WRAPPING UP THE INTERVIEW DAY

The interview day usually flies by quickly, so it's no surprise if you still have some questions at the end of the day. Not to worry; many residents are happy to give you their pager or home phone numbers and talk with you at greater length after hours.

If you really want to learn more about the program, but cannot stay longer because of other scheduled interviews, speak to the departmental secretary or a house staff member about possible arrangements for a return visit. This will allow you to spend more time on rounds, in clinic or surgery, in conferences and in the surrounding neighborhood. In addition, it will give you an opportunity to confirm or modify your initial impressions of the program.

Be sure to jot down your impressions of the program while they are still fresh in your mind. After you have visited four or five programs, the details will start to blur together. To keep your facts and impressions straight, write down all your thoughts about a program as soon as you can at the end of the day. Use the program evaluation worksheet provided (Appendix C) if you need something to organize your thoughts. You will thank yourself later

DON'T GET LURED INTO BASHING OTHER PROGRAMS.

WRITE DOWN YOUR THOUGHTS ABOUT THE INTERVIEW VISIT RIGHT AWAY.

when you can rank your programs with organized notes while your class-mates are banging their heads against the wall trying to remember which program had the deluxe call rooms with the well-stocked refrigerators and HBO.

## FOLLOW-UP LETTERS

Unless your interviewer explicitly tells you not to do so, write a letter to thank the program for its hospitality and to express your continued interest. This typed letter should be composed and mailed no more than a few days after the interview, while memories of the interviews (on your part and theirs) are still fresh. The sincere follow-up letter can help solidify the impression you left on the interviewer before it is washed away by subsequent interviews.

Personalize the letter by mentioning a specific topic that was discussed during the interview. You can also use the letter to update your application file if you recently received any honors or awards. The letter should be addressed to your interviewers. Do not be shy in stating why you liked the program and that you will be ranking it highly—if you plan to do so (See Figure 9–1). If you are a strong applicant who wants to attend a less competitive program because of personal reasons, share them with the interviewer. Keep in mind, however, that the NRMP urges you as a general rule not to tell programs how you are ranking them. Finally, most interviewers will not mind a phone call for follow-up questions, although if you do not have an urgent reason or a specific question for one of your interviewers, follow-up calls to programs can appear pushy.

A THANK-YOU CARD INSTEAD OF A LETTER IS A NICE PERSONAL TOUCH IF YOUR HANDWRITING IS NEAT.

**FIGURE 9-1**

January 21, 2000

John Alpha, MD, PhD
Best School of Medicine
123 Fourth St.
Heartland, USA 12345

Dear Dr. Alpha,

I would like to thank the university for making my visit so pleasant. I especially enjoyed our discussion regarding the future of health care reform. I agree that though current measures are wholly inadequate, they are at least a step in the right direction.

I was very impressed by the program's commitment to urban health care and by the dedication and enthusiasm evident in the house staff and faculty. I plan to rank your program highly, and I hope that you will keep my application in mind. If you have any other questions, please do not hesitate to call me at 415-555-5555.

Sincerely,

Jane Beta

Specific reference to interview.

Tell them why you like the program in honest terms.

Express enthusiasm without committing.

Example of a follow-up letter.

# The Rank List and Match Day

## HOW DO I RANK THE PROGRAMS?

Ranking is an important part of the Match process, not to be taken lightly. Year after year, really smart applicants do really stupid things when it comes to ranking programs. Once and for all, there are two rules, and **only** two rules, to keep in mind when you set up your rank list.

**Rule #1—Rank programs in order of their desirability.** After you have visited all the programs, reviewed your notes, and have weighed all the pros and cons, list the programs in order of their desirability. Enter the programs on your rank list in this exact order. The object is to match with your most desirable program, not to match with your first ranked choice. Do **not** rank a program lower because you believe your chances of attaining that program are slim. Do not rank a program higher because someone said that you were at the top of the program's rank list (see below). Ideally, the programs at the bottom of your rank list will serve as backups—acceptable programs that are a sure bet.

**Rule #2—Rank all acceptable programs.** After you have completed your interviews, you should have only two categories of programs: acceptable and unacceptable. **Do not rank any programs that you wouldn't want to work in.** Remember that you are under contract to report to the program where you match. If the program is on your rank list at all, you're telling the NRMP that you are willing to go to that program if you match there. You are under no obligation to rank every program that you visit. You must decide, however, whether it is better to match at a less than ideal program or to take your chances in the Scramble if you do not match. The latter option, though highly undesirable, is certainly viable in specialties that have a large number of unfilled positions on Match Day, such as anesthesiology.

The two rules we have given you do not guarantee a match, they guarantee only that you will do the best you can do with what you have to work with (Table 10–1). If you are having a tough time putting all your information together, walk through your rank list with your significant other, friend, or career adviser.

| Table 10–1. Ways to improve your chances of matching. |
| --- |
| • Realistically assess your competitiveness and the competitiveness of the programs. |
| • Apply and interview at a sufficient number of programs. |
| • Rank all programs acceptable to you. |
| • If you aim for a tough specialty, have a backup. |

## The NRMP Matching Algorithm

The same algorithm is used by the Canadian Residency Matching Service (CaRMS). Outlined below is a simplified explanation of the NRMP algorithm. Your *NRMP Handbook* describes the steps in greater detail.

1. The process begins with an attempt to place an applicant into his or her first choice program. If a match cannot be made because the program is already filled or the applicant was not ranked by the program, then an attempt is made to match the applicant with the next program on his or her rank list. This process continues until a tentative match is made or the applicant is left unmatched.

2. In the next round, an attempt is made to place the next applicant into his or her first choice program. If this new applicant is more attractive to a program than another applicant who is already tentatively matched, the least preferred applicant is removed to make room for the more desirable applicant and a new tentative match is made. The process will repeat for the candidate who was removed from the match.

3. The process is carried out for all applicants until each applicant has been tentatively matched to the most preferred choice possible or all choices have been exhausted.

4. When all applicants have been considered, the tentative matches become final and the process is complete.

In short, each applicant moves "down" his or her rank order list (ROL) until a tentative match is made or all choices are exhausted, while each program moves "up" their ROL. Note that no applicant can be bypassed by a lower-ranked applicant for a certain program. If the higher-ranked applicant did not tentatively match there, it's because the applicant already had a more desirable offer in hand. Since the algorithm was computerized in 1974, the process takes only minutes to run.

## Is the NRMP Algorithm Fair?

The NRMP matching algorithm has worked well since the 1950s and has survived largely intact. However, there have been some recent questions raised about its fairness. This debate was featured in 4 articles in the June 1995 issue of *Academic Medicine*.

In these articles, groups such as the American Medical Student Association, the Public Health Citizen's Health Research Group, and the Medical Student Section of the American Medical Association advocated that the matching algorithm be changed given its supposed bias towards residency programs at the expense of applicants. In May of 1997, in response to this controversy, the board of directors of the NRMP voted to replace the existing matching algorithm with a new applicant-favorable algorithm beginning in 1998. An article in the September 3, 1997 issue of JAMA discusses the effects of the change in the NRMP matching algorithm.

The authors of the article compared the results of the old and new matching algorithms on the ROLs submitted by all applicants and residency programs in the 1987 and 1993 through 1996 NRMP matches. The differences in matches produced by the two algorithms was small: fewer than 0.1% of applicants would have received a different match and most, but not all, of the applicants would have done better with the new applicant-favorable algorithm. About 0.5% of programs would have received a different match and most, but not all, would have done better with the former NRMP algorithm. With both algorithms, applicants and programs were most likely to receive their preferred match by submitting ROLs based solely on their true preferences rather than strategic behavior.

**Bottom line.** Is the NRMP Match algorithm unfair? More importantly, will it affect you? At one in a thousand odds, it is extremely unlikely. And with the new algorithm, these odds are even less important. Should you worry about it? Probably not. You are much more likely to get hurt by a poorly thought out rank list than the current match algorithm.

## How do couples rank programs?

The *NRMP Handbook* includes a step-by-step guide for creating a couples rank list. The advice is generally sound. You and your partner should first rank programs as if you were matching on your own. Turn to "How do I rank the programs?" above for guidelines. Then, you should list the possible program pairs if you are ranking more than one program in the same city. In addition to program pairs in the same city/area (Type 1), there are 2 other types of program pairs to consider: pairs of programs not in the same city/area (Type 2) and combinations in which one partner goes unmatched (Type 3). Consider creating and ranking Type 2 pairings if separation is tolerable. These pairs allow both partners to match semi-independently. Because Type 2 pairings are not restricted by geography, the number of possible permutations is large. Consider creating and ranking Type 3 pairings if it is acceptable for one to match and the other to enter the Scramble. This is usually preferable to both of you going unmatched.

Ranking the program pairs is a classic process of give-and-take. Fortunately, the process can be less painful if you and your partner have communicated well during the application process, and thus have a understanding of each other's preferences. Couples must decide how much weight to give the location versus the programs. Regardless, the process may take a few evenings. After all, your rank list can easily be over a hundred pairs long. When ranking Type 3 pairings, factor in the location; it will be easier for the unmatched partner to scramble in a large city with many training programs. You can register for the couples match when both of you enter your couples list.

## Supplemental Rank Order Lists

When an applicant ranks an advanced position (which begins 15 months after the Match), he or she also submits a ranking of PGY-1 (transitional or preliminary) programs on a Supplemental Rank Order List (SROL). The applicant can submit more than one SROL, thus tailoring PGY-1 preferences depending on the location of the advanced training. If you do not match into an advanced position, then your SROLs will not be used. If you go unmatched on your SROL, your advanced match result still holds. You can rank up to 15 programs on your SROLs combined at no charge.

THE ALGORITHM CONTROVERSY IS A TEMPEST IN A TEAPOT.

RANKING A COUPLES LIST IS AN EXERCISE IN OPEN COMMUNICATIONS AND COMPROMISE.

PROMISES MEAN ZILCH
UNLESS IN WRITING FROM
THE RESIDENCY DIRECTOR.

## "We are ranking you at the top of our list" (Not!)

Programs often send candidates follow-up letters after the interview to affirm their interest. Sometimes they will assure you that you will be ranked at the top of their list. This may be a pleasant compliment; however, do **not** count on it, and do **not** let it affect your ranking of their program. Even if they say this, it simply means that you can match no lower than that program. Some applicants have an instinctive but unfortunate tendency to favor programs that they believe are more likely to take them. Other applicants allow these follow-up letters to limit the length of their rank list inappropriately. Again, all acceptable programs should be on your rank list.

## Under-the-Table Deals

In some of the most competitive fields, program directors or department chairs often call applicants after the interview but before Match Day to ask the applicant about his or her ranking of the program. **It is a violation of Match rules for programs to ask you for this information.** Your ranking of programs should have absolutely no effect on a program's ranking of you. Unless the caller represents your top choice, the question is only a golden opportunity for you to hang yourself. If you tell the program you are not ranking them first, they might drop you on their rank list to ensure that they get their top picks. Believe it or not, some programs would rather minimize how low they go on their rank list instead of just going for their top candidates. If you receive such a call from one of your top choices, **get a commitment in writing from the residency director.** If they balk, then all bets are off. Otherwise, consider telling them that you expect to rank them #1 or very highly even if you are not. After the Match, consider reporting this violation to your Dean of Students, the NRMP or the appropriate specialty board.

## Entering Your Rank Order List

As of the 1999 Match, all rank order lists for specialties which participate in the NRMP Match must be submitted electronically through the Internet using the Rank Order List and Input Confirmation System (ROLIC). You will indicate your preferences among the programs at which you interviewed. Programs entered in the ROLIC system may include preliminary or transitional, categorical, advanced programs or a combination of these. You can also list several different specialty types (e.g. internal medicine, family practice, surgery, etc.). If you rank advanced (PGY-2) positions on your Rank Order List and wish to also secure a first year (PGY-1) position, you will also be required to submit a Supplemental Rank Order list. More detailed information can be found in the NRMP Handbook for medical students or on the NRMP website (http://www.aamc.org/nrmp).

Students applying to specialties that have their own match must send their rank list to their specific matching program. Contact information for these specialties is provided in Chapter 1.

Turning in your rank list can feel like asking someone to marry you. You're absolutely sure until the moment you turn in that piece of paper. Then you start thinking, "Wait a minute. Did I do the right thing?" But it's too late; you have already sent the list. Most of the soul-searching and turmoil focuses on the order of your top three choices. Hold on to your list until you can think this through. Discuss strengths and weaknesses of these three programs with your significant other or a close friend. Is it too late to modify the rank list after you have turned it in? Well, actually, no. The NRMP will accept faxed changes for a few days after the deadline has passed, if your Dean of Students makes a request on your behalf. But because exercising this option is disruptive and depends heavily on your dean, don't view it as an opportunity to allow you to mull over your rank list past the deadline. **Use this option as a last resort only.**

## MARCH MATCHNESS ("IT'S AWESOME, BABY!")

The NRMP Match itself is run in late February. The results are known to your dean's office several days before Match Day, which is usually on a Wednesday in mid-March. The Monday or Tuesday before Match Day is the moment of truth for most. If you do **not** hear from your dean's office during this period, you can assume that you matched. If you fear the worst, you can call your dean's office or the NRMP 2 days before Match Day to learn if you matched. If you did, then you must wait until Match Day itself to find out where you matched. If you do learn that you did not match, please read on for information about the Scramble.

A list of matched independent applicants by code is published in *USA Today* on Unmatch Day (the day before Match Day). If you are an independent candidate and your code is **not** listed, call the NRMP after 9 AM (EST) to confirm your match status.

At medical schools on Match Day, the results are announced simultaneously across the nation at noon, Eastern Standard Time. Many schools organize ceremonies or more casual breakfasts around this event; applicants often bring their significant others to provide moral support and to share in the anticipation. The atmosphere is usually electric by the time the signal is given to open the envelope.

PRANK CALLS FROM CLASSMATES PRETENDING TO BE FROM THE DEAN'S OFFICE ARE NOT FUNNY.

## WHAT HAPPENS IF I DON'T MATCH? THE SCRAMBLE

If the news is bad, the fact that you did not match does not amount to a personal rejection from the entire medical profession. It might help your bruised ego to recognize that failure to match is most often due to a poorly thought-out rank list or simply applying in a small competitive specialty. It might also be comforting to know that you are not alone: about a thousand U.S. medical students and several thousand non-U.S. medical student applicants enter the Scramble every year; most of them find quality residency positions immediately.

For better or worse, you'll have to postpone your moping and self-pity till later. You will be apprised of your situation by your dean on Unmatch Day or the day before. You will also be given an *NRMP Results* book that lists programs in your specialty with unfilled positions. You may be able to meet with your adviser or your department chairperson, who can review the NRMP results and quickly draw up a "hot" list of programs for you to pursue. In many cases, your adviser or department chair will intervene and contact program directors on your behalf. **Note that you are not restricted by specialty.** Many applicants decide to pursue additional programs in another spe-

NOW IS NOT THE TIME TO PANIC!

THE RANK LIST AND MATCH DAY

195

cialty because there are too few Scramble positions available in their initial specialty selection (eg, surgery).

If your adviser is unavailable, or if you are not a U.S. medical student, then you will have to contact the programs directly. After you make your list of programs in order of interest, then track down the program phone numbers in AMA-FREIDA or the Green Book. You can also look up the area code of that program and call information, (area code) 555-1212, to get the local number. You will then need to assemble the following documents for a faxable application file:

► Dean's letter
► Transcript
► A copy of the NRMP Universal Application
► Your CV
► Any letters of recommendation that you may have

Begin your quest by calling programs in the order in which they appear on your "hot list," starting at noon EST on Unmatch Day. The day will be hectic and stressful; steel yourself for busy signals and harried program secretaries. You will have to make a conscious effort to remain calm and friendly. You will need to fax your application file to interested programs. Your dean's office or the department in your specialty should give you full access to their phones and fax machines. Positions will be offered by phone. If you are offered a position at a program that is low on your "hot list," ask them how long they are willing to hold that position for you. Otherwise, be prepared to wrap up your acceptance over the phone. Most unmatched seniors are placed within a day.

**THE SCRAMBLE BEGINS AT NOON EST ON UNMATCH DAY.**

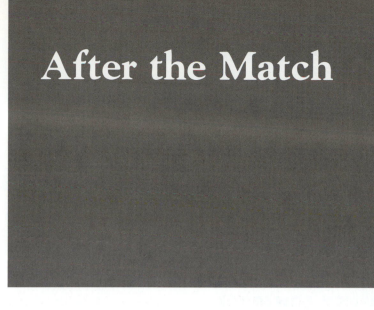

# After the Match

**11**

## THE DAY AFTER

The aftermath of Match Day is not unlike the day after an election. Even if you're ecstatic about the outcome, you can't just party for a week; there are tasks to be performed, such as gearing up for your new position and thanking your supporters. You want your new associates to be glad they "elected" you. So shake off the hangover and . . .

Call your program, first of all, to introduce yourself in an enthusiastic manner as one of the incoming interns. Ask for the "class" roster; chances are you'll know a few of them either from your school or from the interview trail. Then find out who the chief residents will be. Inquire about scheduling. Are there any electives? Will you have any say in balancing easy and tough months? How are vacation days assigned? This is also the time to mention any non-negotiable schedule constraints, such as your upcoming wedding. In addition, ask what information or credentials they would like from you. Some of the more academic programs have some prerequisite reading before the program begins. It's also important to ask about their ACLS/ATLS training policy. Some programs expect you to come with certification in hand; others will put you through an ACLS course when you start.

After your introductory contact, write thank-you letters to the program director and to your interviewers. They were your advocates during the rough-and-tumble ranking sessions. When they receive letters from you, they will be assured that they made the right choice. Plus: don't forget to thank your advisers and all those at your school who supported you with letters of recommendation. They would like to know where their support landed you. Take the time to give them honest feedback so that they can adjust their advice for future students.

## WHAT IF I'M NOT HAPPY WITH MY MATCH RESULT?

The good news is that over 80% of U.S. seniors will get one of their first three choices in the Match. Even if you did not match at one of your top choices, however, you should have few regrets if you followed the two cardi-

> **IN MOST INTERNSHIPS, YOUR SCHEDULE IS YOUR LIFE.**

- Resident's responsibilities
- Salary and other stipends
- Other benefits
- Length of contract and terms of renewal
- Policies for sick leave, parental leave, etc.
- Grievance and sexual harassment policies

"IF YOU CAN'T BE
WITH THE ONE YOU LOVE, LOVE
THE ONE YOU'RE WITH."

nal matching rules outlined in Chapter 10. First of all, be reassured that feelings of insecurity are a normal reaction to major life decisions. This case of the jitters is commonly known as "buyer's remorse." Our advice is to relax; the feelings should pass. Secondly, remember that your participation in the NRMP Match means at least a 1-year commitment to the program.

## THE RESIDENCY CONTRACT

After the Match, you will receive a residency contract to sign and return to your program. The Accreditation Council for Graduate Medical Education (ACGME) recommends that certain terms and conditions be clearly addressed in the contract (Table 11–1). Before you sign your contract, **understand the definitions of all essential terms**.

You will also begin receiving a large number of forms to fill out from your residency program. Try to stay on top of these forms to help insure a smooth transition into your internship. You will most likely receive a vacation request form and an elective request form. Remember that your vacation weeks will usually be during your elective or outpatient rotations, so think about when you may want to schedule a lighter month or when you may have to travel (i.e., wedding, graduation ceremony). You will need certain documentation that you may want to organize into a file. Items such as proof of citizenship (birth certificate, passport, social security card) and ACLS/BCLS certificates are useful to have on hand. You will probably also need to provide a headshot (you can use your ERAS application picture) for your residency program's composite.

## LOANS

It is a good idea to get a handle on your student loans now, so that you will not have to spend as much time thinking about them during your busy internship year. Most U.S. medical schools' financial aid offices will conduct "exit" interviews where they will provide information, resources, and strategies for dealing with your loans. Come to this interview prepared: know your loan types and amounts, lender, interest rates, loan features (i.e. grace period, deferment, capitalization). The more prepared you are, the easier it will be for you to understand and plan your repayment options with your financial aid officer.

## GETTING SET UP

Moving right along . . . your next set of priorities is relocating. Nobody enjoys the process, but it doesn't have to be the mother of all battles either. Some choice pointers:

## Housing Tips

Housing should be arranged before graduation if at all possible. First: Explore the pros and cons of renting versus buying; housing costs vary widely across the United States, and a good deal for one area may not be your best bet in another. Often it's best to talk to the current house staff at your program about their impressions of the local market. As long as you can afford the payments, buying a small home or a condo may make investment sense if you plan to stay in the area for several years. On the other hand, renting will give you the flexibility to look for bigger and better places after you have a chance to size up the area. For the first year, it's safest to focus on finding a short-commute, hassle-free situation, as every hour is precious during internship.

There are many ways to find housing opportunities: (1) Call up friends who live near the program for housing tips; (2) Ask the residency office about housing options; (3) Visit a realty service or a professional rental service; (4) Go to the local library to look at the classifieds section in local newspapers or use the Internet to search for available housing in your new city. Listings available through rental and roommate agencies tend to be of higher quality since the listing fee is self-selecting. Unless it's a huge hassle, plan to visit the city for at least 2 to 4 days to find and finalize housing arrangements.

## Moving Tips

In anticipation for your move, prepare change of address cards and arrange mail forwarding with the Post Office. For tracking purposes, you should make a catalog of your belongings (if you have a lot of material you might organize it by room) and photograph valuable items for insurance purposes. Selling or donating all non-essential belongings will streamline the move and your life in the long run. In addition, make sure you have adequate packing materials before you start the job (Table 11–2). If you are on a tight budget, boxes can usually be harvested in waste disposal areas behind the hospital. Boxes for IV bottles have dividers and are perfect for glassware. Alternatively, many grocery stores or liquor stores will donate their large cardboard boxes that are sturdy enough for packing books. Furniture stores are typically more than happy to supply you with large sheets of leftover plastic and bubble wrap.

You have several options for moving your stuff once it's packed. If you have little or no furniture (or none worth taking), then your moving will be easy. Just pack your nonbreakable belongings and call UPS at (800) PICK-UPS for a pickup. UPS does have a limit on the maximum size and weight per box, so call for details. The company automatically insures goods for up

---

**TABLE 11-2. Packing essentials check list.**

- ☐ Packing boxes
- ☐ Newspapers
- ☐ Plastic/bubble wrap
- ☐ Cord/rope
- ☐ Packing tape
- ☐ Scissors
- ☐ Utility knife
- ☐ Markers
- ☐ Labels

to $100 per box and sells insurance for belongings of greater value. Move your valuable or more fragile items personally.

If you have furniture worth keeping, then you might want to move it yourself. There are a number of self-moving companies with one-way moving vans, like Ryder and U-Haul. If you contact a local branch of such a company rather than the central office, you can often bargain for the truck/van rental. This is the cheaper way to move; however, beware of the hassle factor. It's worth considering hiring professional movers to do the job; it costs more, but you'll avoid piling the stress of moving your belongings on top of starting your internship.

## Settling Down

By all means, take a vacation; but give yourself at least 1 or 2 weeks to settle into your new home before the start of internship. You will need this block of time to set up your household, open bank accounts, turn on utilities, and install a telephone line. If you wait to show up 2 days before a very busy internship begins, it may take you the next 2 months just to unpack. Extra time will also give you a chance to explore the neighborhood and city before internship takes over your life. You won't want to waste time later locating grocery stores, affordable restaurants, 24-hour gas stations, and the like. Try to streamline all non-medical aspects of life (e.g., bill paying, shopping) so that your time off is "quality time."

## LICENSING

The Match is over; you've moved into a nice apartment five minutes from the hospital. Now all you have to do is brace for internship, right? Wrong. During the throes of internship, you will have to apply for **licensure,** the **USMLE Step 3,** and **DEA registration.** Unfortunately, these applications require you to fill out a mountain of paperwork and involve such things as notarized documents, fingerprints and birth certificates. Thus, the preparation you begin **before** starting internship will minimize your stress and vastly enhance your ability to become licensed when you want to be or are required to be.

The tips on the following pages were provided by Licensure Unlimited to help you get started. Licensure Unlimited is a professional service that specializes in managing application processes for physicians. Armed with this information, you will be able to control all three of these critical processes so that you can become licensed in a timely fashion with a minimum number of surprises (e.g., deadlines, exam dates, and required fees). Alternatively, if you desire additional assistance, you can contact Licensure Unlimited at:

Licensure Unlimited
4023 Lincoln Ave
Culver City, CA 90232
(800) 838-1979

## What Is Licensure?

"Licensure" is the legal term that denotes approval to practice medicine. It is granted by a governing body on the basis of the laws in your jurisdiction.

Some states offer several types of licensure—e.g., training, military, inactive, *locum tenens*, temporary, or permanent. Periods of licensure also vary from state to state; some licenses are valid for only one year, others for two. Similarly, some licenses can be renewed after a set period of time that is based on your birthdate, while others are renewable on an annual basis during a particular month of the year. All 50 states require that applicants have successfully passed the USMLE Steps 1, 2, and 3 exams to be eligible for licensure. This entire process typically costs roughly $1500.

You should also be aware that in some states, the medical board can fine residents and programs up to $2500 for failing to obtain licensure as defined by the law. In support of this legislation, some programs have even been known to terminate house staff who fail to become licensed by state-mandated deadlines.

You should also remember that medical boards process thousands of applications each year, usually on a first-come, first-served basis. They will **not** process files that are out of order **for any reason whatsoever.** So be courteous when discussing your application with licensing technicians, and allow for plenty of time.

Most residents will also want to avoid using their vacations for completing applications—although the latest information indicates that approximately one-third of all residents nonetheless wait until the midpoint of their internships to begin reviewing issues surrounding licensure.

Once you have matched, we recommend that you obtain the regulations for licensure in the state where you will be training. Then carefully review those regulations, paying particular attention to USMLE Step 3 exam dates and deadlines, when you are eligible for licensure, and when you are required to be licensed in your jurisdiction.

## Steps Toward Licensure

The following tips will help further your goal of obtaining licensure in a straightforward and timely manner. Contact the state board before internship to obtain licensure information. Once you know the deadlines, start the licensure application process **six months** before the licensure deadline in your state. Before you Perma-Plaque or frame your medical school diploma, be sure to make 10 copies of it on 8 1/2- by 11-inch paper. Send all forms via certified, registered or express mail, or enclose prepaid postcards to allow for acknowledgment of materials received. When dealing with medical board personnel, be very courteous (they're just like residency application secretaries: cross them and you're history) and honest about your background.

## The Nitty Gritty

Table 11–3 summarizes the most common materials requested by state medical boards for licensure. Once you know what is required for licensure in your jurisdiction, you can prepare for the application process by doing some or all of the following, as appropriate:

- ► Identify the location and cost of **photographic services.** Be sure to find a photographic service near your place of work, as you may need to make a couple of visits there during work hours.

DO NOT MAKE YOUR NEED TO BE LICENSED AN EMERGENCY FOR THE MEDICAL BOARD.

- Medical school diploma (either original diploma or an official copy with the registrar's signature and school seal)
- Official medical school transcript
- Official undergraduate school transcript
- 2 to 3 recently taken passport photographs
- 2 to 3 letters of recommendation
- Letter from residency program director
- Official USMLE Steps 1, 2, and 3 score reports
- Fingerprints
- Completed application with notarized signature
- Application fee (usually around $600–$1000)
- Letter of good standing from any other state licensing boards that you were granted licensure from

▶ Identify the location and cost of a **notary public.** If there is no notary public in your facility, try real-estate offices or banks. Be aware, however, that many notary publics have limited hours of availability. Also be sure to complete your application before obtaining notarization, but **do not sign the application** until you are in the presence of the notary. A valid picture ID will also be required—e.g., a driver's license or a passport.

▶ Identify the location and cost of fingerprinting services.

▶ Identify potential personal references, and then contact them to discuss their willingness to serve as references on your behalf.

▶ Research the addresses and costs of obtaining academic transcripts.

▶ List all hospitals and addresses where staff privileges have been granted.

▶ Order a certified copy of your birth certificate.

▶ If you have changed your name, locate and obtain documentation that will verify that change.

## Obstacles to Licensure

Potential obstacles to licensure that **both U.S. and international medical graduates** may face are as follows:

- **Missing critical deadlines (e.g., failure to apply for and take the USMLE Step 3 in conjunction with licensing deadlines.)** Since one of the primary requirements for licensure is successful passage of the USMLE Step 3 examination, you must time the Step 3 exam so that you take it at least three months prior to your licensure deadline. This will allow for the scoring of your exam as well as for the reporting of your scores to the medical board. Another benefit of taking the exam early is that it allows you time to take it again should that prove necessary.
- **Failure to include correct licensure/exam fees along with your application.** Most medical boards will return your application if the fees you enclosed are incorrect. You should also be aware that most application fees are nonrefundable.
- **Failure to provide complete and accurate information on your application.** In reviewing your application, medical boards sometimes uncover discrepancies such as inconsistently reported attendance dates. If this is the case, the board must write you a letter explaining the discrepancy they found and what you must do to rectify it.

- **Incomplete documentation.** As is the case with all bureaucracies, forms are not always completed properly by other institutions. Unfortunately, however, incomplete forms sent to the medical board by your undergraduate school, medical school, or training program will be returned to you to correct. You may then need to call the facility where the error occurred to ensure that the forms are properly handled the second time around.

- **Submitting unrequested documentation to the medical board.** Documents that have not been requested but are enclosed with your application can confuse and frustrate licensing technicians. Moreover, the inclusion of such documents in your application package can raise troubling questions both about your application and about your ability to follow basic instructions.

- **Administrative holds on transcripts.** Transcripts can be held for a variety of reasons, including delinquent student loans, unpaid library fines, and the like.

- **Administrative holds by training programs.** Program directors may deny your request to complete your licensure form on the basis of incomplete patient chart dictations, etc. (This is rare, but it has been known to occur.)

- **Disregarding requests for additional documentation.** Requests for additional documentation by the medical board are commonplace but should not be ignored, as some states consider a file closed if it has not been fully completed within a certain period of time. Thus, you should provide all documentation requested in a timely manner.

- **Failing to report a change of address to the medical board.** Most states will not forward licenses in the mail. Thus, if you have recently moved, be sure to notify your medical board of your new address **in writing** at the earliest possible time.

- **Failing to keep copies of documents that are submitted to the medical board.** It is always a good idea to keep extra copies of all forms and their addresses. That will help you track lost documents while also helping resolve questions the board might have on a particular document.

- **Exhibiting abusive behavior toward medical board personnel.** Medical board personnel typically have a very large workload. Thus, working cooperatively with them is clearly in your best interests. Remember, board personnel don't make the licensing laws; they're just chartered to uphold them.

- **Starting the application process too late.** If you are not licensed by the deadline set by your state medical board, you may be unable to continue your training program.

The following potential obstacles to licensure apply to **international medical graduates** (IMGs) only:

- **Getting forms completed by a foreign medical school.** Documents sent to foreign medical schools often require additional processing time. It can thus be highly advantageous to have someone living near your medical school oversee the process of document completion, mailing, etc.

- **Failure to complete sufficient hours in required clinical rotations.** IMGs should carefully review licensing requirements for the state from which they are requesting licensure.
- **Inadequate documentation of individual clinical rotations.** Some states have their own individual forms to be used for documenting each rotation. Again, contact your medical board for details.
- **Failure to use medical-board-approved translators for documents written in other languages.** Some state medical boards have a list of translators whom they have deemed acceptable for translating application documents. Contact your medical board for more information.

## First Aid for the USMLE Step 3

As of December 31, 1999, you may no longer use the Federation Licensing Examination (FLEX) components or the former NBME certifying examinations to fulfill eligibility requirements for Step 3. To apply for Step 3, you must meet the following requirements before submitting an application:

1. Meet the Step 3 requirements set by the medical licensing authority to which you are applying.
2. Obtain the MD degree (or the equivalent) or the DO degree.
3. Receive a passing score on Step 1 and Step 2.
4. If you are an IMG, obtain certification by the ECFMG or complete a "Fifth Pathway" program.

In addition, most states will also require that you have completed or have almost completed one year of postgraduate training in a residency program accredited by the ACGME.

When you send in your application for Step 3, you are unable to select a time period within which you wish to take the exam as you did for Steps 1 and 2. Instead, allow 4 to 6 weeks for the processing of your application. When this is completed, a scheduling permit will be sent to you. You may then call a Sylvan Technology Center to schedule a test date. Step 3 is available throughout the year except for 2 weeks in January. It is a two-day examination that must be taken on consecutive business days; therefore, it is important to both schedule your test date as soon as you receive your scheduling permit and to keep your appointment. As with Steps 1 and 2, Step 3 uses computer-based testing. For general information on licensure and Step 3, contact:

Federation of State Medical Boards (FSMB)
Department of Examination Services
400 Fuller Wiser Road, Suite 300
Euless, TX 76039-3855
(817) 571-2949
http://www.fsmb.org

Be sure to plan ahead for the USMLE Step 3. Although the cost of taking the exam is currently $485, some states add administrative charges to this overall cost. These extra charges can, moreover, vary from state to state, since some state medical boards conduct the Step 3 examination themselves while others rely on the USMLE to do so. The application for Step 3 also differs somewhat from those for the USMLE Step 1 and 2—e.g., your signature must be notarized, and additional documents may be required. You can use Express Mail, Federal Express, or UPS to deliver your application, but faxed documents are unacceptable. Be sure to make copies of all documents, and keep in mind that it takes six to eight weeks to score the exam. The following are some basic administrative guidelines to follow in preparing to take the USMLE Step 3:

- **Contact FSMB or call your state medical board for a USMLE Step 3 application, and read it carefully.** Experience has taught that it is critical to verify when you are eligible to take the Step 3 exam, as this may vary from state to state.
- **Start the application process early.** Begin pulling together your supporting documentation as soon as possible.
- **Find out when your state requires you to be licensed and whether that date differs from that of your training program's requirement.** To help you determine when to take Step 3, work backward from your state licensure deadline to determine when you should schedule the exam. Be sure to factor in the six to eight weeks that it will take for scoring and notification of results.
- **Locate a photographic service for required application photos.**
- **Identify a notary public in your facility to obtain required notarizations.**
- **Oh yeah, don't forget to study.**

## DON'T FORGET TO WRITE

Congratulations! You've made it to internship. We hope that the advice and information in this book was helpful. Much of what you have read comes from the experiences of students who have gone before you. We hope that you'll share the lessons you have learned with those to follow, by e-mailing us or sending in the contribution forms in the front of this book. As for internship, nothing can save you from that. But don't worry—in a year, you'll be done (or done in). Best of luck.

## REFERENCES

Federation of State Medical Boards (FSMB) website (http://www.fsmb.org). Medschool.com website (http://www.medschool.com).

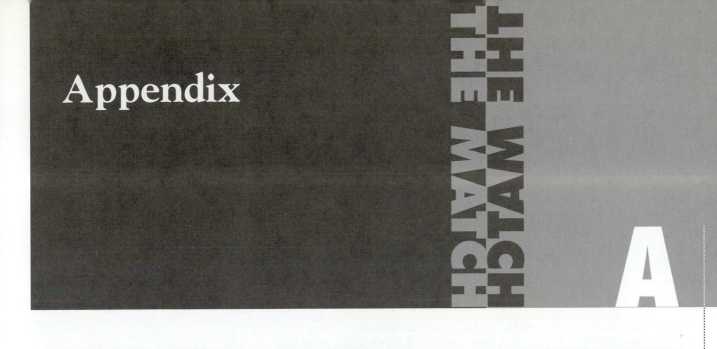

# Appendix

| Commonly asked interview questions by specialty.[1] | |
|---|---|
| **Specialty** | **Commonly Asked Questions** |
| All specialties | Why did you apply to this program?<br>What are you looking for in a residency program?<br>Why are you interested in this specialty?<br>Where do you see yourself in the future? |
| Anesthesia | Why do you want to enter anesthesiology?<br>Why did you apply to our residency program?<br>What do you envision yourself doing after you finish your residency?<br>What other residency programs are you applying to, and why did you choose to apply to these programs? |
| Dermatology | Have you had any prior research experience in this field?<br>What is your potential contribution to the field? |
| Diagnostic Radiology | Why do you want to enter radiology?<br>Why did you apply to our residency program?<br>What do you envision yourself doing after you finish your residency?<br>What other residency programs are you applying to, and why did you choose to apply to these programs? |
| Emergency Medicine | Why have you chosen a four year program vs. a three year program (and vice-versa)?<br>Why are you interested in emergency medicine?<br>Tell me about an interesting case that you have seen.<br>What are some of your personal strengths and weaknesses?<br>What would you do for a living if you couldn't go into emergency medicine? |
| Family Practice | What is your focus in family practice?<br>How do you feel about specific ethical issues in healthcare, such as end of life issues?<br>Do you feel comfortable with working with patients of all ages? |
| General Surgery | Do you enjoy working under pressure?<br>Have you done any research in general surgery?<br>Tell us about an interesting clinical case that you saw during your general surgery rotation. |
| Internal Medicine | What are your personal strengths and weaknesses?<br>We're going to give you a clinical scenario and you'll provide the diagnosis. |
| Neurology | What research projects are you involved in?<br>Could we have your opinion on an ethical issue? |
| Neurosurgery | What research projects are you involved in?<br>Ethics questions may also be asked. |
| OB/GYN | What was the most interesting case that you saw as a medical student during your OB/GYN rotation?<br>Have you done any research in OB/GYN? If so, tell me about your research project. |

---

[1] Reproduced with permission from the Medschool.com Community website (http://students.medschool.com).

| Commonly asked interview questions by specialty. (continued) | |
|---|---|
| **Specialty** | **Commonly Asked Questions** |
| Ophthalmology | Will you answer some clinical questions?<br>Do you have any contingency plans?<br>What is your research/clinical background? |
| Orthopedic Surgery | Why do you want to enter orthopedics?<br>Why did you apply to our residency program?<br>What do you envision yourself doing after you finish your residency?<br>Have you done any research in orthopedics? If so, tell me about your research project. |
| Otolaryngology | What are your academic and research interests?<br>Where do you see this practice heading in the future? |
| Pathology | What are your post-residency plans?<br>Why have you chosen this field? |
| Pediatrics | Do you react well with children and their parents?<br>Why did you decide to go into pediatrics? |
| Physical Medicine and Rehabilitation | What is your focus in physical medicine?<br>Do you feel comfortable working with patients of all ages?<br>What are your personal strengths and weaknesses? |
| Radiation Oncology | Are you comfortable handling issues related to death and dying?<br>What are your thoughts about euthanasia?<br>(May present a clinical scenario around the ethical issues of euthanasia.)<br>What are your personal strengths and weaknesses? |
| Urology | Have you done any research in urology?<br>Tell us about an interesting clinical case that you saw during your urology rotation.<br>What are your personal strengths and weaknesses? |

# Index

*Page numbers followed by t indicate table. Page numbers followed by f indicate figure.*

**NOTES**

Ms. Shonbrun (Anne)    (Assis Reg)
    (718) 270-4552
            -1107
visitstudent @ downstate.edu